Rethink

Reshape

Redefine

*Desire * Determination* Discipline* & Dedication

Dennis C. Simmons

Rethink Reshape Redefine

Dennis Simmons

Dennis C. Simmons
2015

First Printing: 2015

ISBN-13: 978-1519190185

ISBN-10: 1519190182

Dennis C. Simmons
Mind, Body and Soul Boot Camp 1
http://www.rejuvgrp.com

dennis730simmons@gmial.com

Contents

Acknowledgements

First and foremost I like to thank everybody for giving me this opportunity to share my knowledge and experience. I was born in the inner city of St. Louis, Mo. I am a very experience, Certified Trainer I have been working out over 20 years I have also facilitates Anaerobic and Aerobic class. I would like to dedicate this book to my mother, Lavern Simmons. I know that she is looking down on me smiling like a proud mother should, knowing that I have made this transition. I would like to give special thanks to my baby brother Dion for the support and the inspiration and for bringing out the best in me and not letting me accept anything less.

DIET HISTORY

One of the first pieces of information to obtain from clients is their diet history. A client should provide at least three days' worth of information, preferably 2 weekdays and 1 weekend. The client should be as detailed as possible to include:

1. What foods are being consumed
2. How much food is consumed
3. When/What time the food is consumed

The 4 D's

DESIRE: YOU MUST WANT IT

DETERMINATION: TO DEVELOP A GOAL
WITH ACCOMPLISHMENT

DISCIPLINE: YOUR MIND MUST BE INTO
SCULPTING A PERFECT PHYSIQUE

DEDICATION: WHEN YOU WANT IT BADLY
ENOUGH

Chapter 1

Knowledge on Proper Exercising

Fundamental technique is the backbone of every fitness program to a safe and healthy workout. Without the perfect technique and form you will not stimulate the intended muscle, in fact you might actually cause injury with little results. I must admit that I have seen a lot of people in the gym that have no idea to properly train their muscles, and this includes even some certified fitness trainers on television. They do not know what they are doing, and the only people that suffer are you, because you rely on the person's wisdom and guidance. I do not want you to read this book once and forget, rather I want you to learn and utilize this knowledge, and continue to want to learn and utilize this knowledge, and continue to use perfect form and technique for great results.

There are two types of training which are unique in their own capacity. You have Anaerobic exercise (e.g. weight training), and Aerobic exercise (e.g. walking, bike riding, etc.). From experience I can say with confidence that these exercises could and should be looked at hand in hand, like night and day, because they complement each other. The anaerobic, which is weight training shapes the body, and also increases your metabolism permanently. Just as weight training reshapes the body, so does fitness exercise, it just does not have the impact or superior look that weight training gives you. On the other hand aerobic exercise keeps you lean and gives you the flexibility needed to compete like a lot of athletes need, as well as stamina.

If you are a professional body builder, you would not want to do a lot of cardio because that will make you lose weight and mass, something you need as a body builder to compete; just as you need to be lean and flexible through aerobic exercise to compete in fitness sports. The type of exercises depends on your need of training or what goals and purpose you have for working out, that what makes the difference.

Now let's discuss the unique techniques for both anaerobic and aerobic exercises, and how you can get the best results from each one or both together. Anaerobic, weight training is best effective in 60 minute sessions that should be the maximum because the levels of muscle, fat burning and testosterone begin to drop, the glycogen that is stored as carbohydrates within your system are the fuel that your muscles use to contract would be depleted. Now that you don't have the hormones to produce muscle growth, continuing to train past 60 minutes will cause impaired recovery that leads to overtraining; and now your body can't recover from its training session.

It is very possible that you would lose strength and muscle mass. As an example, have you ever been in the gym working out with someone when they say. "Man, it seems like I am not getting any stronger or bigger?" Does that sound familiar? That is what happens when you over train. Aerobic exercise is the cornerstone of any fat-burning within its fat-burning zone.

To determine your fat burning zone you must use the following formula; [Fat-burning zone=220 – (your age) x 0.75. 50 and 40 year old men have approximately 135 heart beats per minute. As long as you are 10 beats from your number you are on target. Aerobic exercises are just like working you abdominals to get the best results from them is to work them out first thing in the morning on an empty stomach to prevent dehydration.

Drink 16 to 24 ounces of water. This is why it's important to do aerobic exercise in the morning time because it burns 300% more body fat than any other time during the day. The body has to go to its fat stores in order to get the energy it needs to complete the activities because the glycogen within your system has burned out because you don't have any stored carbohydrates at that time. This is why it takes 20 to 30 minutes for aerobic exercise to start burning fat because that is how long it takes the body to deplete its glycogen (stored carbohydrates) and switch to burn fat.

Then it takes an additional 20 minutes, but you can work out for at least 90 minutes with aerobic exercise. If you weight train first, then go to aerobic exercise for 20 to 30 minutes for the body to deplete its glycogen.

By following these simple workout guidelines, you can get a perfect physique by using the combination of both types of exercises at the proper times and proper durations. Your workout depends on your purpose. If you are going to become a professional body builder then you would want to do 20 to 40 minutes, three times out of the week without weight training on those days because you do not want to lose mass.

Core Strength

Flexibility, stability and core strength are very important to a training program. A lot of times it is overlooked by trainers. When muscles are tight it limits muscles ability to contract properly movement. That wills likely cause injuries and the opposing muscle to contract improperly because no muscle works by itself. This is why many back and hip injuries are related to weak core muscles. Stability is critical for everyone because it promotes balance. If the core is weak it cannot functionally properly. This will cause muscle imbalance; as we get older our stability and balance is compromised, they will degrade if not addressed. Training the core (mid-section) consist of dynamic movements that will gravity the center and isometric exercise. Medicine ball, physic ball, balance boards sit ups and hyperextensions are great tools to train the core.

Physical Fitness

What is physical fitness? Physical fitness is having the energy and the strength to perform daily activities after a workout. Also your heart, lungs and muscles should be strong. For body fat the range for women should not exceed 25% of their body weight. For men fat should not exceed 18% of their body weight. Fitness measures within four (4) parts:

Cardio Respiratory

Muscle Endurance

Muscle Strength

Flexibility

There are two (2) categories of endurance, cardio respiratory and muscle endurance is defined as "the ability to keep moving for long periods of time with a steady rhythm. Whatever method you chose to use anaerobic or aerobic you have to understand the function that it will be demanding; within your goal of time frame. Personally I think anaerobic and aerobic once again goes hand and hand rather you are competitive in a specific sport of function as a peak training athlete this is how you stay ahead of the game. It's easy to race through a set. If the weight is heavy, you get psyched and want to punch it through the roof on each rep. If the weight is light, you get into a groove and "pump out" your reps like you're dancing to a club beat. While both methods do allow you to move the weight from point "A" to point "B" neither fully stimulates your muscles because you're using momentum. To promote muscle and strength, keep the tension on the working muscle. Studies have shown that sets lasting between 40 and 70 seconds are best for achieving muscle growth. Shorter reps imply heavier weights, so those are best for pure strength. Longer sets, naturally, would benefit endurance goals.

Variation

You can fall into a rut by adapting to your program, variation is very important in working out. Resistance training or aerobic training using different exercises. Rep range requires your body to new motion pattern and muscle sequence. Research has shown that the body starts to adapt to any strength training plan within 3 to 4 weeks. Strict isolation is a physiological impossibility but focus on long periods of the same, exercise could be considered isolated to the muscle, but no muscle can contract on its own; without the assistance of at least one total separate muscle group. You can make imbalance to any muscle group, if doing the same thing for a long period.

Aerobic training session typically last 15 to 60 minutes, depending on current fitness level. With the average duration falling between 20 to 30 minutes. Aerobic intensity level is very important toward a desire goal by simply monitoring your heart rate with the karvonen formula. This is commonly used by trainers:

220-age (in year) - maximum heart rate

Pulse for 15 seconds *4 = rest heart rate*

Rest heart rate + (0.60 * maximum heart rate- rest heart rate) ex HR

General Exercise

FAT LOSS:

Fat loss can be achieved in different ways. One organized method is circuit training. You perform one set each of several exercises back – to-back with no rest in between. This keeps your metabolism stoked so you burn calories at an accelerated rate. In addition it saves time.

Lower reps with heavier weights, higher reps with lighter weights. Heavy weights attacks your system harder, activating more muscle than lighter set and requiring more calories to be burned in order to fuel them.

FATIGUE:

Exercise is supposed to make you feel better and infuse you with energy, but initially you may experience bouts of fatigue after your workouts. This fatigue is part of the body's adaptation to the new exercise make some people feel like they've made a wrong decision because they should feel better. How much fatigue you experience, and whether you experience it at all, depends on your choice of exercise. Those who start at a $1/2$ a mile walk won't get fatigue. They tend to feel better, but those who choose to take on a jogging or a cycling program where they're going to work out at a moderate intensity may feel more fatigue. The key to avoiding the wall of fatigue is to start slowly and progress in small steps.

Fitness and fat burner

Circuit training based on compound movement performed 4-5 total sets selected exercise with a pushing movement a pulling movement and a leg press or squatting movement. Now these, movements should be consecutively until completing 4- 5 circuits. Circuit training with heavy exercise should not be performed by beginners. However a more experienced weight trainer should proceed with caution. When planning total sets for different muscle groups or circuit training, the size of the muscle group play a major role. Which will determine the number of used sets because the smaller size the fewer total set and the larger the size the greater to the damage muscle target.

Fear of strength training

A common statement used by women; "I don't want to get big or bulky." Guess what ladies? Developing of bulging muscles and loss of femininity will not come over night, without really trying for it. Focus on cardio does increase percentage of body fat with a weaker muscle that will cause some injuries. Strength training will not only cause development beautifully feminine and athletic physique; nut balance your overall fitness level.

Weight loss and weight gain

Research has shown that 70%- 80% of people that loss weight within a 2 or 3 year span has gained that weight back. Not only did they gain that weight back that they lost, but gained more back than before. It has been proven also that a lot of retired professional athletes, body builders or typical workout people gain a lot of weight not just because they just stop working out. That do have a great sufficient part to gain weight back. But they continue to keep that intake calories regiment, they are used to doing when they were working out.

Unfortunately, when gaining weight the body distributes fat uniformly throughout the body. Now you are at the mercy of your genetic background that will determine rather the fat be evenly or unevenly within your frame. Fortunately you loss it with that same concept. But remember when losing weight or gaining muscle, the recommendation rate is 1 pound per week any faster will cause fat accumulation.

Chapter 2

Things You Should Know About Nutrition & Weightlifting

The formula:

Each day- no matter what foods you eat you should take in roughly 15 to 20 percent protein. 20 to 25 percent fat and the rest carbohydrates. That means that well over half of everything you eat is high-carbohydrate food. Yes, protein is the key nutrient for repairing and growing muscles, but chances are that you are already getting to much protein. If you eat more protein than the body requires, it either flushes it out of the system or uses it as fuel. In fact, it hurts your energy levels.

No food or nutrient endows you with bigger muscle. What builds muscle is training and hard workouts. Within your genetic.

Before lifting, eat an easily digestible, high carbohydrate, low protein snack. This way you'll have some extra glucose floating about in your bloodstream for energy, and you may reduce muscle tissue damage from lifting.

Carbs break down in the body to form glucose and glycogen, sugars that provide energy. Insulin, a hormone, enables the muscle cells to convert glucose into glycogen, and store it until it is needed.

Make carbohydrates the central food of each meal and snack, and you'll have more energy staying power and intensity in your work-outs.

Don't stuff. Don't starve. Eat small, frequent meals. Do this to keep your energy level stable and your caloric intake more even. You get the calories you need and not a lot of excess. This encourages your body to use them as muscle fuel rather than to store them as fat. Carbohydrates are more important than protein. You don't need more protein. Carbohydrates fuel your workouts and provide you with ready energy.

Carbohydrates

Carbohydrates are made up of the elements carbon, hydrogen and oxygen. There are two basic kinds of carbohydrates- the starches, called complex carbohydrates; and the sugars, or simple carbohydrates. Those consuming a high-carbs, low protein diet ended up leaner than those on a high protein diet.

The best way to store your metabolic furnace is not by taking hormone pills or shots, but by stepping up your activity. Carbohydrates are primary source of fuel in the human diet, which should consist of 58% of the body's total caloric intake in healthy individuals.

Simple carbohydrates or simple sugars are primarily in foods that are very sweet, such as fruit juices, syrups, honey, molasses and the majority of the processed food in the industrialized diet.

Complex carbohydrates are found in whole, unprocessed foods such as fruits, potatoes, corn, rice and most vegetables. Complex sugars in food are stored as starch or glucose polymers. Our bodies break down the complex sugar into mainly glucose in order to digest it and absorb it and then assimilate the sugar into a complex storage material called glycogen which is found primarily in the muscle tissues and liver. There are four calories per one gram of carbohydrates. Glucose is the most abundant sugar in the body.

Load up on carbohydrates; Banish all notions that starches stick to the ribs. Carbohydrates burn fastest of all the bodies energy sources, and aren't easily converted into fat. When they are converted, the process itself burns calories. On top of that, carbohydrates spark the release of adrenaline, which burns still more calories. Carbohydrates just cause the metabolic machinery in the body to turn over faster.

Fiber

A high fiber diet fills you up without filling you out, keeps you regular, helps lower your cholesterol level, and may help reduce both your blood pressure and your risk of colon cancer, along with other health benefits.

Nutritionists advocate getting at least 20 grams of fiber per day. Two apples a day will give you between 18 to 35 daily grams of fiber. You can also get fiber from whole-grain breads and breakfast cereals, brown rice, strawberries, pears, and various vegetables, especially ones with edible stalks and stem such as broccoli and carrots.

Proteins
Basic Fundamental Facts;

- Proteins are found in various foods such as animal flesh, organ meats, eggs, dairy, nuts and seeds, and various combinations of grains and legumes.

- Proteins are made up of amino acids. There are 22 amino acids, and 9 of these are essential in the diet.

- One gram of protein equals 4 calories.

- 12% of the diet should be proteins.

- One pound of fat yields 3500 calories of energy.

- A high source of energy yielding 9 calories per 1 gram of fat.

Cut back on protein
Your body needs protein for building everything from muscle to bones. Unfortunately, it doesn't need as much as most of us give it. "The average American eats twice the protein he needs." An excess of protein can make you feel heavy, sluggish, and over time, physically feeble. For optimal health, eat 1 gram of protein for every 3 pounds of

body weight per day, so that would be about 50 grams for a 150 pound man.

You are what you eat

When eating eggs use whites for low calorie sources of protein. In salads made with hard-boiled eggs it's easy to leave out the yolk. If you have to use the yolk try to limit your yolk to three of four a week.

Chicken, turkey and fish- which contain less total fat and less saturated fat than beef or pork- are preferred sources of animal protein. In any case, keep portions small. A 3 ounce serving is more than enough for most adults.

Your body is a machine, it will run as well as its fuel allows. You do not need to give up everything you love to eat in order to protect your health, but you do have to learn to practice discretion and moderation in your food choices.

Moderation also means portion control emphasis on some foods, and less on others. Start thinking about how to make sensible selections within the framework of basic four. Of the various possibilities in each category, choose those foods that are lower in fat, especially in saturated fats lower cholesterol, lower in added sweeteners, and lower in salt. In making such choices you will necessarily increase the amount of fiber and complex carbohydrates in your diet. You will probably also reduce the number of calories without even trying too.

<u>Evolutionary Change</u>

If you make the changes too abruptly you're likely to resent them, and you'll probably build up cravings for various beloved foods you've banished from your menu. On a per-pound, your requirements for protein declines with age. Pound- per pound, infants need nearly three times as much protein as adults.

You must consume "complete" protein within the same meal for your body to get full value from the protein you eat. Most animal proteins are "complete", whereas most vegetables proteins are "incomplete". However, two or more incomplete proteins can be combined in a meal to form complete proteins, or tiny amounts of complete proteins can be used to supplement an incomplete one. In a T-bone steak, about 20% of the calories are protein; with the remaining 80% as fat. At the very best, an extremely well-trimmed T-bone steak will still contain 50% of its calories as fat.

Chicken is also a lean source of protein. The quality of the protein is as good as steak, but without skin 64% of the calories in chicken are protein, and 31% are fat. Thus, ounce-for ounce, chicken provides more protein than steak, but steak has two and a half times as many calories, and twice the amount of fat.

In whole milk, protein is 21% of the calories, and fat provides 48%. Skim milk (all the butterfat removed) is 40% protein and 60% carbohydrates.

Whole wheat bread is 16% protein, 80% carbohydrates. Oatmeal is 15% protein and 70% carbohydrates.

Peanut butter is loaded with good things like protein, fiber, vitamins, and minerals; nevertheless, the problem some guys mistakenly have with peanut butter is the fat content- which is sky high. It is healthy, monounsaturated fat, the kind that is okay to eat. Peanut butter, which contains a lot of, vegetable oil, is 17% protein, 13% carbohydrates, and 66% fat.

Vegetarian

Some vegetarians are strict vegans, which means they consume no animal sources of food including, dairy, meat, fish and eggs. Some vegetarians will eat dairy and fish. If they are strict vegans, they need to supplement vitamin B12 and possibly iron, if they are female. They should pay close attention to their protein intake. It is important for them to get them complete proteins from their diets. If vegetarians are a novice, a good protein powder may be beneficial. Most vegetarians get enough protein from the diet to meet adequate requirements if they eat a balanced wholesome meal.

Caffeine

Caffeine has an ergogenic effect in more ways than one. Not only does caffeine stimulate the adrenals for action, but it circulates fatty acids for fuel during a workout (Black Coffee).

PEANUT BUTTER

Peanut Butter is loaded with good things like protein, fiber, vitamins, and minerals; nevertheless, the problem some guys mistakenly have with it is the fat content – which is sky high. But it is healthy, monounsaturated fat – the kind that's okay to eat.

How to use the nutrition information with recipes

Bodybuilder like to intake a lot of protein for repairing and growing muscle, carbohydrates for energy and keep their body fat down. As you age your total daily calorie intake should be about 60 percent of carbohydrates, 25 percent of fat, and 15 percent of protein because too much protein can hurt your energy levels because the body will use it as fuel. To convert these targets into grams, multiply your daily calorie need by the targets, and then divide the carbohydrates and protein products by 4 and the fat product by 9. For example, the calculations for an active man who need about 3500 calories per day follow.

60% carb x 3500 calories= 2100 carb 4/=525 gram carb 25% fat x 3500 calories = 875 fat calories 9/=97 gram fat 15% protein x 3500 calories = 525 protein calories 4/=131 gram

The body works best when you ingest food in certain combinations, many guys ask me for advice about what and when they should eat. The muscles require a supply of blood during working out, when you get the pump that experience is from blood swelling up your muscle. If you eat too much before training your muscle will suffer because the digestive system will use excess amount of blood to digest a big meal. So you could take up to 2 to 4 hours before you training after eating a heavy meal but 90 minute will do but it could take all the way up to 6 hour for your stomach to empty its content. The following order within the system of digesting its food first; carbohydrates, protein and fatty food are the last to leave.

Hitting Protein & Carbs

Below are the Top Ten sources of protein and carbohydrates for Heavy Weights:

Eat Protein for Strength (One –third of diet):

Lean Meats   Yogurt
Poultry   Nuts
Fish   Beans
Tofu   Skim Milk
Cheeses   Lentils

Eat Carbohydrates for Endurance (Two- third of diet):

Potatoes   Lentils
Breads   Cereals
Rice   Beans
Pasta   Corns
Fruits   Peas

Top Foods to Eat For Tight ABS

Lean Meats and Proteins:
Poultry
Beef
Fish
Egg Whites

Vegetables and Fruit that have Fiber:

Spinach   Raspberries

Collards Strawberries
Kale Plums
Broccoli Carrots
Mellon's
Blueberries

Legumes:
Almonds
Soy Nuts
Quinoa
Black Beans

Whole Grains:
Whole Wheat
Brown Rice
Barley
Bulge

Six Basic Nutrients For Health

Food is more than just fuel that stops your hunger. Food contains nutrients essential for maintaining optimal health and top performance.

There are 6 types of nutrients:

1. **Carbohydrates-** are a source of calories from sugars and starches that fuel your muscle and brain. Carbohydrates are the primary energy source when you're exercising hard.
2. **Fat-** is a source of stored energy (calories) that is burned mostly during low-level activity (e.g. reading and sleeping) and long-term activity (e.g. long training runs and gentle bike riders).
3. **Protein-** is essential for building and repairing muscle, red blood cells. Protein from food is digested into amino acids.
4. **Vitamins-** are metabolic catalysts that regulate chemical reaction within the body.
5. **Minerals-** are elements obtained from food that combine in many ways to form structures of the body.
6. **Water-** is an essential substance that makes up about 60 to 75 percent of your body weight. Water stabilizes body temperature, carries nutrients to and waste away from cells, and is needed for cells to function. Water does not provide energy.

Chapter 3

Maximize Your Growth

Researchers found that growth-hormone release was greater when the subjects performed the additional lighter set after their heavy sets, rather than training heavy alone. That's significant because the higher your level of growth hormone, the greater your potential for muscle growth.

Recuperation

You train because you want to get big, and essentially the muscle-building process occurs in the following three-stage sequence: Stimulation, Recovery and Growth. The stimulation stage is accomplished by putting a training stress on the body. Then begins the recovery phase. Once the recovery phase is complete, muscle growth occurs. Only after muscle growth has taken place is it time to train those particular muscles again.

Overtraining (Symptoms & Cures):

1. General feeling of tiredness
2. Irritability
3. Trouble sleeping
4. Loss of appetite
5. Joint aches
6. Nausea and Light headed
7. Not being in a positive frame of mind

I realized that improvement is enhanced not by training harder and longer, but by training smarter. Think smart and recuperate to accumulate.

5 major factors that affect training

Level of fitness - is based on one's history of exercise. Obviously, the more total hours of training the greater the results.

Intensity- is a much overlooked component of training. To break old records and realize one's potential, the exertion level or intensity must be raised another notch.

Duration- Can affect training in two ways. For anaerobic training, exercise should not last no more than 60 minutes. Optimal levels of hormones fall drastically if intense exercise last 75 minutes. For aerobic training, exercise duration must last at least 20 minutes continuously for aerobic effects to occur.

Frequency- of exercise should be fairly high for training, ideally 4-5 times a week for consistency of adaptation.

Genetics- play a big role in one's potential and should be considered when planning long term goals.

Chapter 4
Guidelines for Repetitions,
Sets & Rest Intervals

Repetitions (reps)—The amount of times that you perform an exercise if you pick up the bar and lower it, pause, and lift it up again; that is one rep. You do the same motion and that is the second rep, and so on.

Sets—A set is a collection of repetition that acuminates in building muscle.

Rest Interval—The amount of time you rest in between sets.

Muscular Failure—The point at which, due to a build-up of lactic acid in the muscle, it becomes impossible to perform another repetition with good form.

Supersets- A combination of exercise performed right after each other without a rest in between.

Guidelines for Reps

For Maximum Strength:

Perform one to four reps per set. If you're going on high- calorie foods, you'll build size; too but increased strength will be the main result. (And strength, in case you don't know, improves your potential to build muscle mass.)

For Maximum Muscle Growth:

Perform six to 12 reps per set. This range is renowned for building pure muscle size. Again, there will be strength and endurance gains as well, but size is the focus.

For Endurance:

Perform 12 to 20 reps per set. If you take part in aerobic sports, sets of 12 to 20 will be useful in preparing your muscle to keep contracting for long periods.

Guidelines for Sets

For Maximum Strength: Three to five sets per exercise

For Maximum Muscle Growth: Four to eight sets per exercise

For Endurance: Two to three sets per exercise

Guidelines for Rest

For Maximum Strength: Rest two to five minutes between sets

For Maximum Muscle Growth: Rest 30-90 seconds between sets

For Endurance: Rest 30 seconds or less between sets

For Fat Loss: Rest 30-60 seconds between sets

Conclusion

Now that we have got the basic knowledge about technique, form and nutrition let us put that knowledge to some use and re-shape our bodies. Remember, technique and form will give you a perfect physical body. But before we get started let me mention one more important thing. Please consult a physician before you start training and when at all possible, exercise with an experienced and qualified trainer until you get familiar on the proper techniques and form. As I like to say, "I'd rather be safe than sorry".

EXERCISE

ROUTINES

Chapter 5
Technique & Form

Technique when working out is very important when it comes to weight training. In this section you will get a basic understanding of the major muscle groups, the exercise to be done to work those muscle groups, and sample workouts for use in working said muscles out. First we will start off by talking about the "chest". Besides the fact that everyone likes doing chest, it is the most fundamental weight-training besides squats. If you had only 15 minutes to train your upper body you would probably do the bench press, and maybe some chin-ups; if you had only 20 minutes to do lower body training you would do squats.

It is always a debate about what the proper bench press grip should be. You have the wide grip, medium grip, and in between grip. The wide grip bench press helps work the outer chest that compliments your lapsed, but you have to be careful because you can injure your shoulder. When using the wide grip do not use heavy weight. Next you have the medium grip which is basically your shoulder length grip. The in between grip helps develop that depth in the center of your chest. Alone with champagne dumbbells, you can the same bench press grip doing incline and decline.

Whether you are doing bench press with barbells on flat, incline or decline, try not to arch your back to much. By arching your back you will improve your bench press poundage, but the advantage is entirely artificial. Also, do not lift your butt off the bench- If you have to do that then the weight is too heavy for you, so decrease the weight.

Another technique or tip to use when bench pressing is the motion and position of the bar. Most people bench press straight up and down. But if you look at the worlds power lifters they push the bar up and slightly at an angle toward the head. This motion is called the J-Lift.

I should also mention briefly the importance of doing proper warms up before doing any workouts on any of the targeted muscle groups in this section.

Dumbbells are something I personally like working out with because it puts mass on your body. It is also good for agilities due to the balancing act requires to use the dumbbells, adding an additional challenge. Dumbbells can be used on the flat, incline, and/or decline bench press as well.

1. CHEST ROUTINE

Flat Barbell Bench:
1 sets of warm ups
4 sets / Reps 15, 12,
10,8

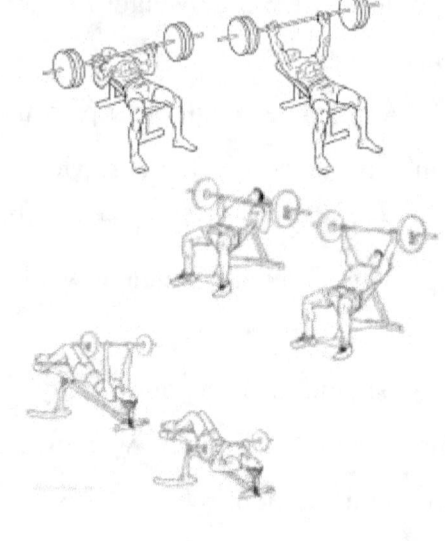

Incline Barbell Bench:
1 sets of warm ups
4sets / Reps 15, 12, 10,8

Decline Bench:
1 sets warm ups
3 sets / Reps 12, 12, 15

Dumbbell Incline Bench:
3 sets / Reps 10, 12, 15

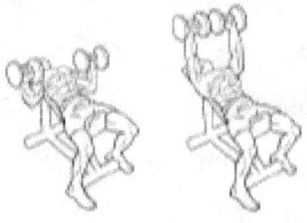

Dumbbell Flyer Incline Bench:
2 sets / Reps 12, 15

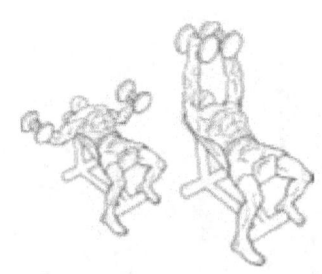

(Find a weight that you can lift)
ALWAYS DO YOUR WARM-UP BEFORE DOING ANY WORKOUT

2. SHOULDERS

Technique is everything when working out. Your shoulder has a three dimensional head including the anterior, medial, and posterior. If you don't learn how to train the shoulders properly then you will not get the right results you desire.

Suggested Exercise

Dumbbell shoulder Press:

This exercise primarily works on the front and side deltoids, with compliments that involve the triceps muscle. Doing the shoulder press, set your bench to a 90 degree angle (in fully upright position), or a shoulder bench that has back support. The dumbbell is supposed to be palms facing in front of you and leveled with the top of your shoulder. Relax your chest while keeping your back totally upright and your head and neck as relaxed as possible. Remember; never turn your head on this or any exercise. When you press the dumbbell at the top don't touch them together, it may cause undue stress onto the rotator cuff muscles, or it might hurt the elbow joint. Slowly bring the dumbbells back down making sure that your arms are wide.

Dumbbell Lateral Raise:

This exercise targets the side deltoids (medial head) by using a lower weight that will allow you to concentrate on perfect form. Stand with a shoulder width stance; slightly bend at the knees to avoid any unnecessary back strain. Hold a dumbbell in each hand with arms down at your sides. Your palms should be pointed towards your body.

It is important that your palms should be facing downward so your shoulder muscles rather than the biceps muscles do the work. Keeping your arms straight and at the sides of your body, lift the weights directly out from the side until they reach the cheeks, and then slowly lower the dumbbell in a controlled fashion back to the starting position.

Military Press:

This is a great exercise to develop all three of the shoulder muscles, but behind the neck presses I do not recommend because you can damage your rotator cuffs. You also can use the exercise with a narrower grip or a wide grip. The narrower grip focuses on the muscles of the medial and deltoids that complement the triceps. The wider grip you go you incorporate the front and medial deltoids. When doing military press make sure that you are sitting upright and your back is straight. Remember, your choice of grip variations determines which certain muscles gets stimulated, so decide what grip you are going to use to develop the overall muscle balance and symmetry of the three heads.

Upright Row:

On this exercise you may use a cambered bar or dumbbell. This exercise helps develop the tie in muscle and trapeziums muscle, as well as the medial head. Doing this exercise you need to be very careful of rotator cuff injuries caused by poor form and excessive weight.

If you are like me, working out in the gym you have seen guys doing this exercise with too much weight , they are swinging, which will cause stress on their rotator cuffs, and put stress on their lower backs. So lighten the weight and use this technique – Keep your back straight and your body still with a shoulder width apart also. Slowly begin by pulling the bar up leading with your elbow to a point where it comes close to your chin. Focus on contracting the muscles of the trapeziums. Lower the bar by maintaining the exact form and posture you did when pulling the bar.

Bent-Over Lateral Raise:

This exercise develops the rear deltoid. A lot of time this muscle gets neglected because people do not make the time to work on this muscle. By doing this exercise you will give your shoulder that fantastic three dimensional look. You can do this exercise several ways. One, by sitting on the edge of the bench, bend at the waist and lift the dumbbell to each side of your body. Another way is by standing and bending at the hip, remembering to slightly bend your knees to take the press of your lower back. This exercise should be done with a smaller weight to get perfect form and rotation.

Military Press:
1 sets of warm-up
3 sets / Reps 15, 15, 12

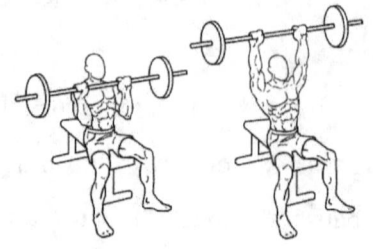

Dumbbell Shoulder Press: 1
sets of warm-up
3 sets / Reps 15, 15, 12

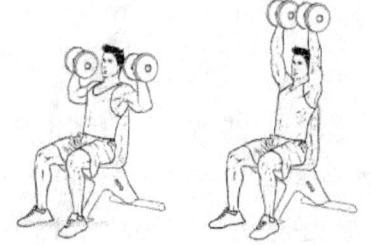

Dumbbell Lateral Raise: 1
set of warm-up
3 sets / Reps 12, 12, 12

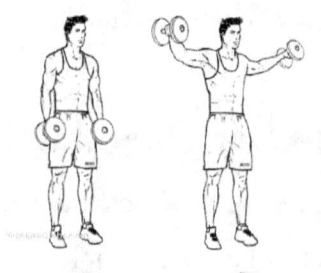

Upright Row:
1 set of warm-up
3 sets / Reps 15, 15, 15

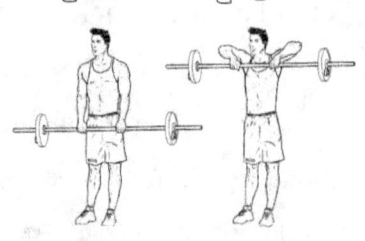

Bent-Over lateral Raise:
1 set of warm-up
3 sets / Reps 15, 15, 12

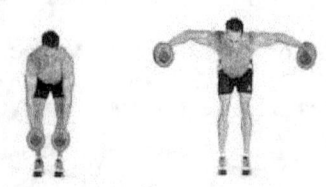

Find a weight that you can lift with perfect form
Do your warm-up sets

3. BACK

The back is composed of several different muscles. The bigger your back is the bigger your chest will be, creating a powerful V-shaped torso, as well as making your waist look smaller. Below are some of the exercises to develop a thicker back that will turn heads.

Deadlifts:

Deadlifts are a unique exercise that helps develop the back. It also helps strengthen the lower back. If you already have a weak lower back try the stiff deadlift. I know you are probably saying, "What's the difference?" Remember; earlier I talked about different variation grips of the bar, angle and feet placement. The deadlifts or stiff deadlifts exercise is about bending or not bending your knees with lighter weight, but the technique and form are the same. Get into a squatting position with the bar centered over the balls of your feet. Grip the bar with an overhand-underhand grip. Pull the bar straight up with your legs and back, keeping it close to your body. As it passes your knees, arch backwards, carefully lower the weight, while keeping your eyes for-ward so you won't hunch over. Find a weight that you are comfortable with because you have to use good form and technique so you won't injure your lower back.

Bent-Over Row:

This exercise with the bar emphasizes the mid-back muscles and latissimus dorsa. Also the lower back, rear deltoids and biceps, so you see this is an overall exercise, but for people that have lower back problems it might be better to use the dumbbell version. Make sure that your knees are slightly bent and pointing directly in front of you throughout the movement. While bending over at the hips make sure that your lower back is not slumped over. Keep your head up and look straight ahead throughout the movement. By doing this you can keep your balance and good posture. When bringing the bar slowly up, stick out your chest while slightly squeezing your shoulder blades. You can also use a reverse grip for this exercise as well.

Dumbbell Row (Lawnmower):

This exercise has less low back involvement. Dumbbell row allows you to focus more on the back muscles because you will be doing one side at a time. This exercise is very similar to bent over rows. Re-member; technique and form is everything in working out. To start find a weight that is light enough to give you a perfect form. Find a flat bench; put your right foot on the floor while your left knee is on the bench, leaning slightly into your left hand to help support your body weight. Your back should be straight and your head up. Bring the dumbbell slowly up, squeezing it and holding it for 2 seconds, focusing to contract the back muscle. Slowly bring the weight down and start the lats.

Wide Grip Pull Down:

This exercise really concentrates on isolating and contracting your back muscles. I have also seen this pull down machine used for behind the back reps, which brings to much stress on your neck and rotator cuff. Any exercise that causes stress or pain, you need to stop immediately and consult with a personal trainer or your physician. After you choose your desire weight, your grip should be twice your shoulder width. Lean back slightly from your hips as you slowly pull down. Stick your chest out keeping your elbows wide. Bring the bar down to your collarbone. You can also use this exercise to strengthen you up for the pull up bar. I would admit that it would be a better back exercise.

Narrow Grip Pull Down:

Doing this exercise keep the palms of your hand closely facing each other. Lean back slightly from the hips while slightly contracting the abdominal muscle for support. Slowly pull down, sticking your chest out while keeping your elbows narrow and close to your body. Squeeze the back muscle for a count of a second or two.

Seated low Pulley Row:

Always perform perfect form because you will avoid lower back injury. To properly perform this exercise make sure that your knees are bent. Try not to lean too forward; a little bit is okay. Sit straight up and plant your feet evenly on the platform. Stick your chest out and retract the scapula and shoulder blades. Keep your elbows close to your body and hand down by your lower abdominals and squeeze.

T-Bar:

The T-Bar is an exercise for the back by bending over onto a shoulder width grip with your feet flat on the platform. Keeping your head straight, slowly bring the bar to your collarbone and squeeze your back together, holding it for 1 or 2 seconds. Remember to bend your knees to avoid stress on your lower back.

Back Routine

Dead lifts:
1 sets of warm-ups
4 sets / Reps 12, 10, 8, 6

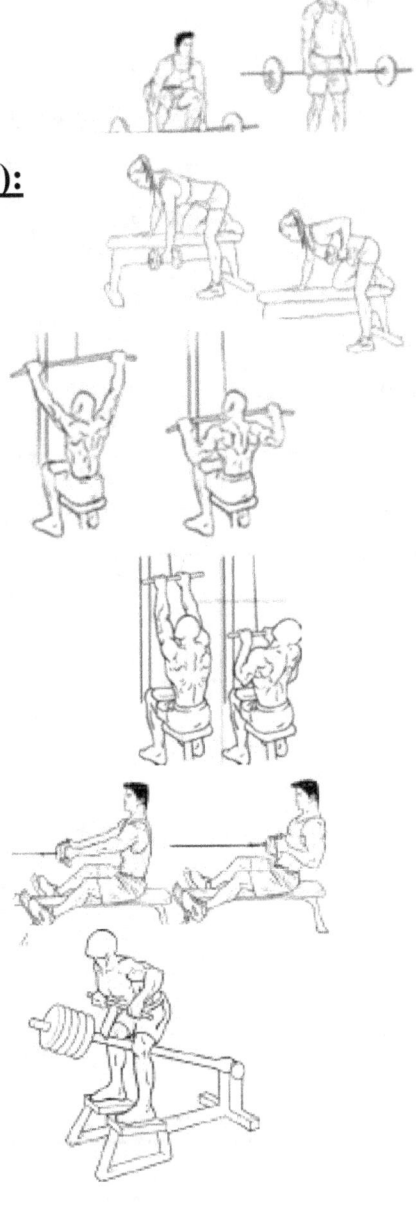

Dumbbell Row (Lawnmower):
1 sets of warm-ups
3 sets / Reps 15, 12, 10

Wide Grip Pull Down:
1 sets of warm-ups
3 sets / Reps 15, 15, 12

Narrow Grip Pull Down:
1 sets of warm-ups
3 sets / Reps 15, 15, 15

Seated low Pulley Row:
1 sets of warm-ups
3 sets / Reps 15, 15, 15

T-Bar:
1 set warm-up
3 sets / Reps 15, 12, 8

Barbell Curl

Doing barbell curls or straight barbell you have to be very careful especially if you are using heavy weights. So, I recommend that you be an experienced person and beginners use lighter weight to avoid stress on your elbows and lower back from swinging the weights, always focus on technique and the proper form. This exercise is a great builder for the entire bicep muscle. Do this exercise standing up, feet about shoulder width apart. Slightly bend your knees so you would not put too much on the lower back, slowly curl the barbell up once you get to the top of the position. Squeeze your biceps hard then slowly lower the barbell back down. Remember; if you are arching your back and swinging the weight STOP! The weight is too heavy, plus that is improper technique as well

Barbell Curl:
1 sets of warm-ups
4 sets of Reps 15, 12, 10, 8

4. ARMS

(Biceps)

Biceps are probably one of the exercises people love to do in the gym. 90%. Most people that train the bicep do so incorrectly with their form used. I will try to explain the proper technique and form to work out the biceps.

Dumbbell Curl

This exercise is a great builder for the biceps muscle. To get proper form choose two light dumbbells. Do this exercise standing up against a wall for good support, feet about shoulder width apart. Slightly bend your knees, and let the dumbbell hang down at your side with your palm and dumbbell facing forward. Keep your shoulder blades squared off and slowly curl the dumbbell up, making sure that your elbows are pointed toward the floor. Once you get to the top of the position, squeeze your biceps hard, and then slowly lower the dumbbell back to the starting position. If you are curling dumbbell and you are arch your back and swing, that means that the dumbbells are too heavy--- STOP! Because, you are putting too much stress on your back, plus that is improper technique.

Incline Dumbbell Curl

This exercise provides a stretch at the bottom of the movement that isolates strict form for the biceps. Remember, technique is your primary focus, so you would use a lighter weight than what you would regularly use for dumbbell curls. Go to an incline bench and set it at a 45- degree angle. This exercise is designed to work the full length of the biceps that complement the outer head of the biceps muscle. We are using lighter weight and are not on an ego trip because that leads to injure.

Use two dumbbells that you can handle using perfect form. Rather than start the dumbbell at your side I usually start the dumbbell on my thighs. Lean all the way back on the bench with your back lying flat on the pad. Grip the dumbbell and allow them to hang at your side, palms facing up. Slowly bring both dumbbells up, keeping your elbows pointed directly at the floor during the entire exercise.

One-Arm Preacher Curl

You can do this exercise on several machines, several different ways. You can use the incline bench, preacher machine, or preacher curl bench. You can also use two dumbbells together or one at a time. This exercise helps develop the lower portion of the bicep muscle that helps develop the ball of the biceps. For whatever choices you make to do this exercise, I do recommend smaller weights that you can control because we want good technique and form. Personally I like using the preacher bench because I am in a snug position with my feet placed flat on the floor. I can concentrate on the ball of the biceps. One arm at a time I bring the dumbbell slowly up and squeeze at the top, curling the weight back down. On the way back down I resist the dumbbell to 45 degree angle because I want to keep that tension of the muscle. Once you have completed your desired repetitions with that arm, switch arms and do that same amount of repetitions on the other arm.

Concentration Curl:

This is a very great exercise for overall development of the biceps muscle. I know this exercise looks like that same thing you were doing with the preacher one arm curl, but you are only concentrating on the ball of the muscle, with this exercise you are concentrating on the whole muscle group. Early on in this chapter we talked about different variation grips. This is one example: To do this exercise you do not curl the weight straight up to your chest, but you curl the weight with your arms angled toward your body. To start sit on a flat bench and bend at the hip, fully extending the arm that you will be exercising while the other arm is resting on your thigh. Slowly curl the weight while beginning to rotate your wrist toward your arm pointing at the ground. Slowly lower the dumbbell down to the starting position. This is one repetition.

Standing EZ-Bar Curl:

The EZ-Bar exercise is very versatile, and is easier on your wrist than using the straight bar. If you have a pending strain such as tennis elbow or tendonitis, I recommend that you do not use the straight bar. Using the EZ-Bar allows you to use both a closed and wide grip curls. These grips here are like opposites that attract because the inner grips (closed) help develop the outer biceps, while the wide grip enables you to develop the inner biceps. Now that we have got acquainted with the EZ-Bar Curl, let's start with the technique and form.

First, decide what grip you are going to work out with. Earlier we discussed about balance and symmetry. Now look at your biceps muscle and see which one needs more work. If you find a weakness or imbalance then address that problem with the proper grip. If there is no noticeable difference, I recommend 2 set of closed and 2 sets of wide grips. Hold the bar across your thighs with your palms facing away from your body. Position your feet, shoulders width apart, bending from your knees slightly back straight as you stick your chest out.

Slowly curl the bar up in an arc-like motion, still keeping your back straight. Squeeze the bar at the top. If you had to swing or arch your back to lift the bar than the weight is too heavy for you. Avoid stressing the lower back. Use a lighter weight as technique and form are the best way to lift weights, and the safest way.

Reverse Curl:

This exercise is done also using the EZ-bar, and it targets the upper forearm muscles. Grip the EZ-bar just like you would for curls, only this time you would hold the bar with palms facing your thigh on the outer handles of the bar for direct forearm stimulation. To prepare this exercise your body should be similar to the way it was with the standing dumbbell bicep curl. So take an overhand grip on the outer handles of the bar. Hold the bar on your thighs palms facing towards your body, standing straight up, feet shoulder width apart. Your chest is out back straight, "no" swinging or arching your back. Slowly bring the bar upward to avoid using the shoulders. Try to contract the biceps muscles while slowly lowering the bar, while making sure your forearms gets that negative resistance. That is one repetition.

This exercise should be done with a lighter weight until you can control it with good form and technique.

Hammer Curl:

The exercise is for the outer biceps, and forearms. The way you do this exercise is standing up, dumbbell with the palms facing each other. You also can do this exercise sitting on a preacher's bench. Bend your knees slightly letting the dumbbells hang down at your side. Keep your body straight, this is the proper posture once you reach the top position. Contract the biceps and forearm muscles, holding as possible for 1 to 2 seconds. Slowly lower the dumbbell to the starting position.

Biceps Routine

Standing EZ-Bar Curl:
1 sets of warm-ups
4 sets! Reps 15, 12, 10,8

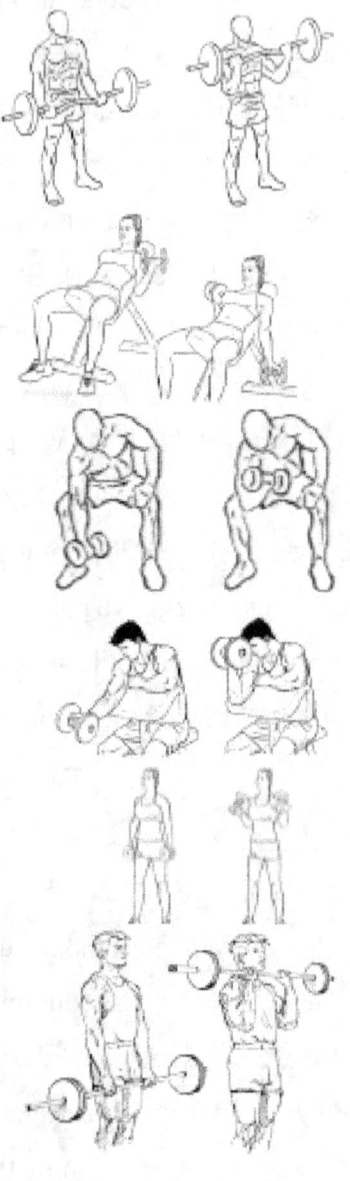

Incline Dumbbell Curl:
1 sets of warm-ups
3 sets! Reps 8, 10, 12

Concentration Curl:
1 sets of warm-ups
3 sets! Reps 10, 10, 12

One Arm Preacher Curl:
1 sets of warm-ups
3 sets! Reps 8, 10, 12

Hammer Curl:
1 sets of warm-ups
3 sets! Reps 12, 12, 15

Reverse Curl:
1sets warm-ups
3 sets! Reps 10, 10, 12

* Find a weight that you can lift with perfect form**
Do your warm-up sets

5. TRICEPS

(Triceps)

The triceps are located on the back of your upper arms, which has a three muscle head like the shoulder. Other similarities with the shoulder are that it requires different angles for a full development. A lot of guys who want big arms focus on biceps, but triceps make your arms look bigger. It also helps your bench out.

Lying EZ-Bar Extension:

To perform this exercise with the EZ-Bar you need to choose a weight that you can control with perfect form. This exercise can also be done using dumbbells, but light in weight. For safety reasons, have someone hand the bar to you after you are lying down on the bench. Place your feet flat onto the floor pointing straight ahead. Lift the bar by pressing it up toward like you are doing a chest press. When you start that is the position you will want to be in to avoid stress on the elbows. Don't start at the bottom with the weight because it creates too much pressure on the elbows and can cause long term injury. Your hand should be 8 – 10 inches apart, your palms and elbows must always face each other during this exercise. As you lower the bar stop just before you reach your forehead, then slowly begin bringing the bar back up to the starting position.

Overhead Dumbbell Extension:

This exercise is performed by using one dumbbell with two hands that targets the middle and inner head of the triceps. This exercise can be done either sitting or standing. I prefer to sit because it helps me focus and isolate these muscles. The important thing about this exercise is your hand grip. If you do not grip the dumbbell evenly, you can create muscle imbalance. To keep from taking all of my focus our attention on getting my hand set evenly, I just put my left thump on my right thumb for two sets, and then I do two more sets with my right thumb over my left. Now, sit on a bench that is 90 degrees, or with good back support because your back has to be flat on the pad. The weight is lifted over your head, with your feet placed flat on the floor. Make sure someone hands you the dumbbell, elbows facing the ceiling, and grip the dumbbell with your choice of grip. With arms and elbows close to your head for triceps isolation, be careful when the weight is over your head. Keep your head straight during the movement. Slowly and staying in control lower the dumbbell to a point where your forearms are slightly below parallel to the ground. As you approach the top of the movement contract the triceps muscle. Do not lock out your elbows.

Triceps Pushdowns:

To do this exercise you have to stay straight as possible with a little slight bent to prevent lower back injury. Stand in front of the cable, take hold of the bar and concentrate on bringing the bar down slowly, pushing while keeping your elbows pinned to your sides as you reach full extension. Avoid locking the elbows joint out hard, but squeeze the triceps muscle as hard as you can. Let the bar come up to the point where your forearm is slightly higher than parallel to the floor. Without resting begin once again.

Bench Dip:

Remember, triceps are 2/3 of the arm, so these bench dips are very important. They can also be done on a parallel bar or in between two flat benches. This exercise helps develop the horseshoe whichever way you choose to do the exercise. To do the bench dip, place two benches parallel to each other so your palms can be on one bench while the back of your feet is on the other. As you lower down, concentrate on using your triceps, toward the ground in a slow and controlled movement until the upper arm and the forearm create a 90 degree angle. Use your triceps to push your back up to the starting position, Remember; technique and perfect form always because you don't want to move up or down in a jerky or uncontrollable manner. Doing that will put stress on the shoulder girdle. If you are going to do triceps dips on a parallel bar you need to be careful for you might think that you are doing chest dips, thus working the chest. So remember the difference between the triceps dip and the chest dips. When you are doing chest dips, bend at your knees and locking your feet, bending forward as you lower yourself. But with triceps dips we are trying to isolate the triceps muscle and avoid stimulation of the chest muscle. Do triceps dips by slowly dipping your body up and down with a straight form.

Triceps Kickback:

This exercise is great, but you have to do this exercise with a lighter weight because you do not want to be sloppy with the form. This exercise should be training one arm at a time, so lean down on a flat bench with the dumbbell in your left hand while your right knees is on the bench. To begin this exercise your upper and lower arm of the triceps should form a 90 degree angle. Once the elbows reaches the point of full extension squeeze the triceps hard, slowly lower the dumbbell back to the 90 degree angle, and avoid hyperextension of the elbow.

Triceps Routine

Lying EZ-Bar Extension:
1 sets of warm-ups
3 sets / Reps 8, 10, 12

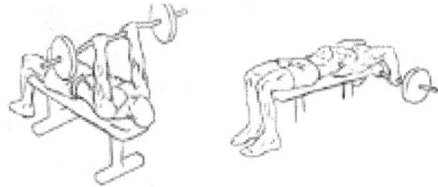

Overhead Dumbbell Extension:
1 sets of warm-ups
4 sets / Reps 8, 10, 12, 15

Triceps Pushdowns:
1 sets of warm-ups
3 sets / Reps 12, 12, 15

Bench Dip:
1 sets of warm-ups
3 sets /Reps 15, 15, 20

Triceps Kickbacks:
1 sets of warm-ups
3 sets / Reps 10, 12, 15

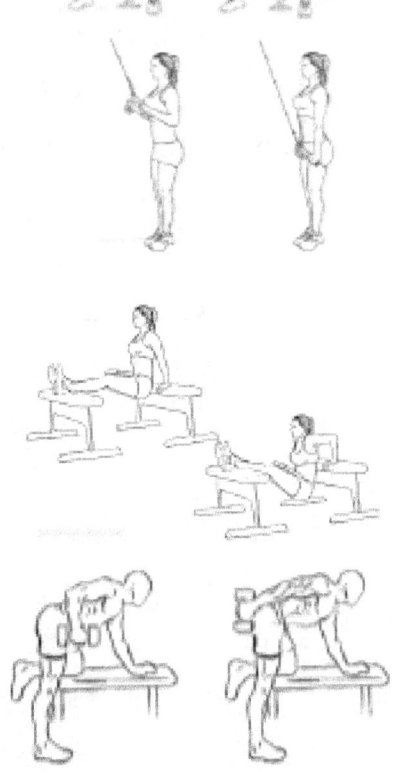

Remember you want perfect technique and good performance, so keep the weight light
Do your warm-up sets to prevent injury

6. <u>LEGS</u>

BARBELL SQUAT:

This exercise help develop the foundation of your body because it incorporates virtually all the body's major group in one way or another. A lot of people that train neglect to so squats for variety of reasons; back problems, don't have time or I will do them tomorrow etc. But building strong ripped legs help balance your upper body, and make you have good posture to stand up straight without a hump in your back. Let's do a test okay, this is how important legs are to the body (example: Get a pencil, sit down at the desk, sit the pencil on the edge evenly on the desk so it won't fall off, now push the pencil a little bit up on the desk and watch it fall, that's because one side weights more than the other).

Now picture your upper body and your lower body that's when you see a lot of big upper guys be leaning over because the upper is too big for their lower, your lower and little legs are not going to be able to support your upper body. Now let's talk about technique and form on how to do a squat with a bar on your back. First just use the bar and make sure that you have a squat safety rack, or in a power cage, the safety bar should be set even with the height of your thighs when they are parallel to the floor. Walk up to the bar and place your shoulder comfortably underneath it and make sure that the bar is on your trapezoid (trap) and not the first and second cervical vertebrae, some people use a pad or a towel, position your hand on the bar with a double shoulder width grip, now put some weight on the bar slowly step back one step at a time, I recommend a spotter because safety is a technique you should consider when weight training, now that you have a spotter let's do some squatting as you take the bar off the rack, step back get comfortable make sure your feet are shoulder width, slightly bend your knees to take some undue stress from your lower back area, always make sure that your knees are pointing directly in front of you. Never let your knees be pass your toes doing squats exercise, always keep your head level at all times and your back straight, if you happen to look down while squatting and the weight is heavy you might jeopardize your safety because you can lose your balance and fall, so you know by now in my book safety, technique and proper form.

DUMBBELL SQUAT:

This exercise performing the same as the barbell, but less stress on your back and better for people with lower back problems, also helps you with your technique and form for the barbell, hold a dumbbell in each hand bend your knees slightly while your palms are facing your body, feet shoulder width apart back straight remember your knees should not go over your feet like you would do with the barbell keep your head leveled at all times and do not drop your eyes because you can lose your balance, also make sure that you do not let your thighs go below parallel because you could injury your low back.

DUMBBELL LUNGE OR BARBELL LUNGE:

This exercise incorporate your buttocks, hamstrings and quads that emphasis on the calves as well, you can also use this exercise with the bar, but if you have problems with your lower back I recommend dumbbell lunge can be done by women and men, but they do require balancing and variation step footing, target different muscle groups, if you place your foot closer to your body you target the quadriceps if you place your foot closer to your body you target the quadriceps, if you place your foot father you stimulate the hamstrings but just like squats you do not want your knees to go pass your toes. Hold the dumbbells in each hand for balance and palms facing the body, your toes pointing straight ahead your knees should be slightly bent to avoid stress on the lower back and from locking the knee joint, step forward with your left foot as you lower yourself until your right foot is 2 inches from the ground, do not forget to let your toes go past your knees slowly, come back up pressing off your left foot without any help from your right, by doing that you are isolating your left leg muscle, and use the right leg for balance.

LEG PRESS:

The Leg press is a great exercise machine, especially if you have a bad back. The leg press has a pad to support your back, what makes the machine so great you can do one leg or two, a lot of people do not let the sled come too far down which depends on your condition. I like the sled to come to the   point just before my thighs would touch my chest because I want the benefits of this depth that the leg press can give me and that works for me. You might have some conditions that won't allow you to go that far. Remember safety and technique are very important. This exercise has a variation of feet placement also if you put your feet high on the platform that less intense of the quad and less knee involvement, lower your foot more tense on the quad contraction but make sure your back and head is on the pad and you are securely in the seat hold on the handle leverage, but don't grip the handle to tightly with the sled slowly come down remember it all depends on your condition how far you bring the sled down.

LEG EXTENSION:

This targets the quadriceps muscles which is the front of the thighs this exercise is excellent to isolation that muscle also recommended by your physical therapist for knee rehabilitation keep in mind about technique and form, the best result with the range of motion you have to lighter the weight besides heavy weight would cause injury to the knee, so your upper leg and lower leg are at an angle which is below 90 degrees, two away to perform this exercise. One or two legs at a time. For both exercises you would get the same result but I believe working one leg at a time is the best because you are able to concentrate on that isolated leg more.

When you are sitting on the machine, make sure you position the back pad so you can be sitting upright, the back of your knee should be against the front of the seat this will help protect the knee, I mentioned earlier about that 90 degree angle that starting position that let your toes be in front of you knees, If you have to adjust the shin pad to the lower point of your shin to optimize leverage plus it helps the resistance to the thigh muscle, you have handles on each side, grip them lightly, slowly lift the weights with your ankles as you get to the top squeezes your quad muscles, your back is supposed to be straight so lean back on the pad once you get to the top slowly bring the weight down at the beginning of the movement.

LYING LEG CURL:

Is for the upper back leg I recommend that you use light weight because heavy weight can make you jerk the weight that will cause lower back problems such as erector spine, it also help the gluteal muscle this a good exercise it can be crucial for over training you can do the same way as the leg extensions with one leg or two legs, but for better isolation on that muscle I use one leg then do the other leg, the reason why I say do not grip the handles to hard because you can change focus on what you are doing also cause the leverage to do the work for you, position yourself on the machine starting with your feet, lay down don't tense up, relax your neck and head, your knees are supposed to be pointed directly in front of you slowly bring the machine to your butt hold for 1 to 2 seconds as you start to go back down slowly control the movement because technique and form is one of our goals.

STIFF LEGGED DEADLIFT:

Remember these are done like you would do dead lift the only different is you want to use lighter weight and keep your knee lock when you dip your hip also it help the hamstring (LOCATED BETWEEN YOUR BUTT) your knees and lower back.

CALF RAISES:

This body part demand a lot of attention because they are very stubborn. The calves are very eye catching just like the abdominals and shoulder, bodybuilder trainers and regular people are conscience are not but, these three areas of the body complement each other that make a person look fit. You need to use different techniques to hit different angles of the calves muscles I know this is the opposite of what I have been saying about heavy weight and high repetition because the activities that you do every day you have to introduce your calves to a training that they are not use to now when you start training your calves we spend a second in the stretched (bottom) position and a second or two in the contracted (top) position.

CALF PRESS:

The Calf Press is an alternative to standing calves raises especially for people that have lower back problems you can perform this exercise two ways, one leg or both legs at the same time. You can get the same results rather you do one or both legs at a time because I can isolate and concentrate on that muscle. Load the machine with the desire weight, your feet should be about 3-5inches apart. Position your feet on the platform so only the upper edge of your foot rest on the platform. The other half will hang off the platform, your leg supposed to be straight with your knees slightly bent, hold on to the handles that is on the side, now raises up onto the tips of your toe as high as you can and hold for a deep stretch, remember technique and form, so do not go too deep on the stretch.

SEAT MACHINE CALF RAISE:

This machine help shapes the calves, to do this exercise you want to have a perfect form rather than just trying to impress people in the gym, so sit down and position your feet in the platform, feet pointed straight place your toes and the ball of your feet on the platform. Lower your heels toward the floor bring the calves to a full stretch, hold for 1 to 2 seconds from this position push from the balls to your tip toe while pushing as high as you can and squeeze, slowly lower your feet back down to an stretch position as you reach the bottom with the heel pointing to the floor do not allow your heel to drop to fast, focus on the stretching of the calf muscle.

The 4 D's

DESIRE: YOU MUST WANT IT

DETERMINATION: TO DEVELOP A GOAL WITH

ACCOMPLISHMENT

DISCIPLINE: YOUR MIND MUST BE INTO

SCULPTING A PERFECT PHYSIQUE

DEDICATION: WHEN YOU WANT IT BAD

ENOUGH

<u>Legs Routine</u>

<u>Barbell Squats:</u>
1 set warm-ups
4 sets / Repetitions 15-12-10-8

<u>Dumbbell Squats:</u>
1 set warm-ups
4 sets / Repetitions 15-12-10-8

<u>Dumbbell Lunge:</u>
1 set warm-ups
3 sets / Repetitions 15-12-10

<u>Leg Press:</u>
1 set warm-ups
4 sets / Repetitions 12-12-15-15

<u>Leg Extension:</u>
1 set warm-ups
4 sets / Repetition 15-15-12-10

<u>Lying Leg Curl:</u>
1 set warm-ups
3 sets / Repetition 10-12-15

<u>Stiff Legged Deadlift:</u>
1 set warm-ups
3 sets / Repetition 12-10-8

<u>Calf Raises:</u>
1 set warm-ups
4 sets / Repetition 15-20-20-20

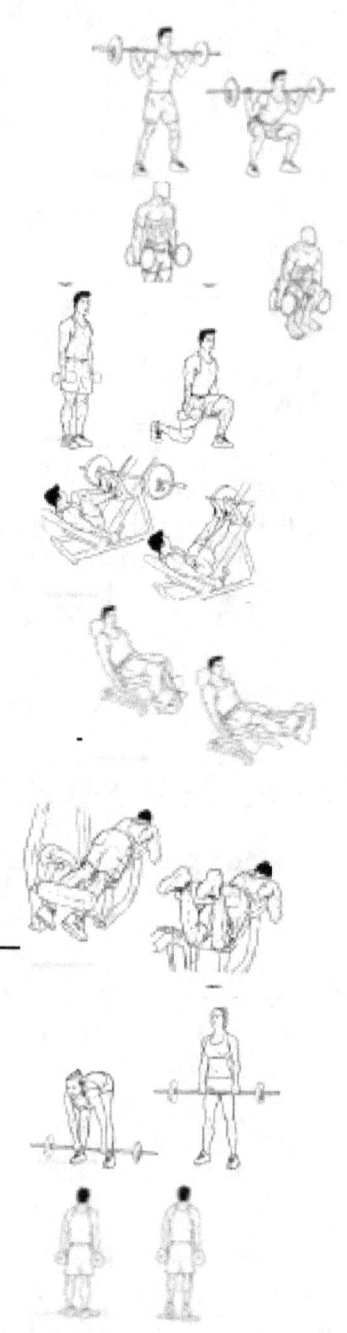

Calf Press:

1 set warm-up
4sets / Repetitions 15-20-20-20

Seat Machine Calf Raise:

1 set warm-up
3 sets / Repetitions 15-20-20

Remember technique and perfect form because you can cause injury to your back, so find a weight that you can perform 6 perfect sets
Don't forget to do your warm-ups

<u>6 Week Program For Beginners</u>

Initially you are going to experience some fatigue doing and after workouts, but that's just part of the body adapting to its new exercise. Circuit training is one method that burn body fat, you perform one set each of several exercise back-to-back with no rest in between. This will raise your metabolism so you burn calories at an accelerated rate, plus it saves time, this routine should take about 25 to 30 minutes that's about the time your glycogen (store carbohydrates) within your system start to burn fat because your energy is deplete with that being the case we are going to go right into aerobic that's how long it will take aerobic to deplete without doing anaerobic there are two great ways of getting results in aerobic one is anaerobic (e.g. weight training). Before you do aerobic the other is first thing in the morning it burn 300 more calories because your glycogen are deplete. Remember before doing aerobics, drink 8 to 12oz of water, to keep from being dehydrated, and always practice technique and good form.

You would do this routine every Monday, Wednesday, and Friday. Every workout day you must rotate a different exercise, but the same muscle group. Always drink water before and after your workout. Do one warm-up set for each exercise.

ANAEROBIC EXERCISE

Muscle Group	Exercise	Sets	Reps
Chest	Flat Barbell Press	1	10
"	Incline Barbell Press	1	10
"	Smith Machine Bench Press	1	10
Back	Bend Over Barbell Row	1	10
"	Lat Pull Down	1	10
"	Straight Arm Pull Down	1	10
Shoulder	Military Press	1	10
"	Dumbbell Press	1	10
"	Bent Over lateral Raise	1	10
Biceps	Barbell Curl	1	10
"	E-Z Bar Preacher Curl	1	10
"	Incline Dumbbell Curl	1	10
Triceps	Overhead Dumbbell Extension	1	10
"	Dips	1	10
"	Cable Press Down	1	10
Leg	Squats	1	10
"	Leg Extensions	1	10
"	Leg Curl	1	10
"	Calf Raise	1	10

In the third week you can go up to 2 set of 10 Repetitions

The second part of your workout is the aerobic (Calisthenics) it is intense for Tuesday, Thursday, and Saturday. Your genes have a lot to do with how your body will respond to training, but there is hope with the right diet and variety of exercise, with many different movements with anaerobic and aerobics you can accomplish a perfect physique with time, some people goals come quicker than others, but do not get dissuade because consistency and repetition will bring you great result along with good technique and form.

50 Jumping Jacks

25 Knee Bends

25 Human Squats

25 Bend Over Toe Touches

30 High Knee Raise (per side)

60 Second Front Plank

30 Second Side Plank

	Sets	Reps
Crunch	2	**12**
Reverses	2	12
Trunk Curl Crunch	2	12
Leg Raise	2	15
Oblique Crunch	2	12 per side
Rope Crunch	2	20
Seated Twist	2	50

6 Week Advance Work Out for Upper body

These exercise should be perform not light or at your maximum but between the two to obtain endurance, strength and burn body fat. So you will do upper body one day then the lower body part the next day. Do one warm-up set for each exercise, rest on Sun-day. If you like you can increase the weights after the third week.

Muscle Group	Exercise	Sets	Reps
Chest	Incline Barbell Press	2	10-12
"	Flat Barbell Press	2	12-15
"	Dumbbell Flyer	2	10-12
Back	Bend Over Barbell Row	2	10-10
"	Reverse Bend Over Barbell Row	2	10-10
"	Dumbbell Row	2	10-10
"	Military Press	2	10-10
"	Dumbbell Press	2	10-10
"	Bend Over lateral Raise	2	10-10
Biceps	Barbell Curl	2	10-12
"	EZ Bar Preacher Curl	2	12-15
"	Incline Dumbbell Curl	2	12-12
Triceps	Overhead Dumbbell Extension	2	15-15
"	Dip	2	15-15
"	One Arm Reverse Grip Pushdown	2	15-15
	BONUS		
Forearms	Wrist Curls	3	15-20
"	Reverse Curls	3	10-15

6 Week Advance Workout for Lower body

These exercises should be perform not light or at your maximum but between the two to obtain endurance, strength and burn body fat. So you will do upper body one day then the lower body part the next day. Do one warm-up set for each exercise, rest on Sun-day. If you like you can increase the weights after the third week.

Muscle Group	Exercise	Sets	Reps
Legs	Barbell Squats	4	10,10,12,15
"	Dumbbell Lunge	4	8,10,10,12
"	Leg Extension	4	10,12,12,15
"	Leg Press	4	12,12,12,15
"	Lying Curl	4	8,12,12,15
"	Seated Machine Calf Raise	4	12,15,15,20
"	Calf Press	4	15,15,15.20
"	Stiff- legged Deadlift	4	8,10,12,15

Program For Heavy Hitters
(Use a three on-one off)
One Warm-Up Set Each

Chest and Back:	SETS	REPS
Incline Barbell Press	4	12.12.10.8
Flat Bench Barbell Press	4	15.12.10.8
Dumbbell Flyer	4	15.15.12.12
Smith Machine Bench Press	4	12 to 15
Cable Crossover	4	12 to 15
Deadlift	4	12.12.10.8
Bent Over Barbell Row	4	12 to 15
Wide Grip Chin-Up	4	15.12.10.8
Seated Cable Rows	4	12 to 15
T-Bar	4	12 to 15
Dumbbell Pull (lawnmower)	4	12 to 15

Shoulder, Biceps and Triceps

	SETS	REPS
Military Barbell Press	4	12.10.8.6
Dumbbell Press	4	15.12.10.8
*Upright Row & Shrugs (Super-Set)	4	15.12.10.8
Bent Over Lateral Raise	4	15.15.12.12
Cable Front Raise	4	15.15.12.12
*Biceps & Triceps (Super -Set)	4	15.12.10.8
Barbell Curl (Straight Bar)	4	15.12.10.8
Dips	4	12 to 15
EZ Bar Preacher Curl	4	15.12.10.8
Two Arm Dumbbell Kickback	4	15.12.10.10
Incline Dumbbell Curl	4	12.12.10.8
Overhead Dumbbell Extension	4	15 to 20
Concentrate Curl	4	12.12.10.8
Cable Press down	4	12 to 15

Forearms:	SETS	REPS
Hammer Curl	4	15.12.10.8
Wrist Curl	4	15 to 20
Reverse Curl	4	15 to 20

Legs:

Dumbbell Lunge	4	12.10.8
Barbell Squat	4	15.12.10.10
Legs Press	4	15.12.12.15
Leg Extension	4	12.12.12.15
Lying Leg Curl	4	15.12.10.8
Stiff- Legged Deadlift	4	15.12.10.8
Donkey Calf Raise	4	15.15.15.15
Seated Machine Calf Raise	4	15 to 20

Abdominals *work every other day*:

Hanging Leg Raise	4	25
Rope Crunch	4	50
Truck Curl and Crunch	4	25
Ball Crunch	4	25
Knee – In	4	25
Side Crunch (oblique)	4	25 per side
Seated Twist	4	25

Chapter 6

Blast Your Chest Routine

If you are a Heavy Hitter and advance in your workout, this exercise is for you. Remember practice good technique and form. This routine is like a circuit training type of exercise, you are going to be lifting quadruple dumbbells by performing one set of dumbbell press, one after the other, then you will start back over by doing champagnes, but first I want you to find a weight with the barbell press that you can do 6 set of 15 reps, then do 4 set of 8 reps with the dumbbell for each exercise a total of 8 set 64 reps (dumbbell) and 6 set of 90 reps with the (Barbell). It's going to be intense so choose your weight carefully, you do not want to go to light to heavy or you cannot perform the exercise. This exercise can be performed with either FLAT, INCLINE or DECLINE benches, you always want to do 1 to 2 sets of warm-up, with this exercise do 1 set of warm-up on the flat bench, then go straight to blasting your chest. If you have 4 dumbbells, let's say 60, 60, 55 and 50 you would bench press them, then start right back with the 65, 60, 55, and 50 and do champagnes for 4 set each for 8 reps each.

Chapter 7

Something for the Beginning Lady's

Briefly I should mention how important it is to use proper form and technique, to warm-up and stretch that muscle before and after you work out, I would like to introduce barbell training for the beginner, so they are challenging those muscles, which will help them balance in their weight lifting training. Remember anaerobic alone will not give you the perfect physique that you see on television or in a magazine. But if you combine a team effort with aerobic and a good nutrition diet plan also with the right supplement within 6 to 8 weeks you will see a tremendous change in your workout that will motivate you to the next level, which is the advance workout by now your technique and form should be incorporated in your workout by using the barbell for 6 to 8 weeks, you have gained strength, endurance, stamina and the "4 D's" Desire, Drive, Determination, and Discipline. Now you are ready to do dumbbells and barbell weight training, also remember to switch exercise ever 6 to 8 weeks because your body get use to that workout. This exercise for anaerobic on Monday, Wednesday, and Friday with aerobic on Tuesday, Thursday, and Saturday, with a rest day on Sun-day. This routine of exercises will define and reshape your body in 6 to 8 weeks.

BENCH PRESS

This could be debatable about the proper technique for beginning with using the barbells or dumbbell press. But for the safety of the trainee let's start off with barbells. Remember doing any kind of resistance exercise you should have a spotter or your trainer. Starting by lying on your back on a flat bench pay attention on how you grip the bar be-cause in that position at the bar that is where you are comfortable with that grip. Do not lift your butt off the bench. To begin with just let's just do the bar because you have some bars that are 25 to 45 pounds and that depends on what kind of bar you are using. Have your spotter to help you take the bar off the rack, feet is planted flat on the floor in-hale going down exhale coming back up, don't forget to breath, a lot of time people bench press and hold their breath, DON'T DO THAT. Lower the bar down to a point just above your chest press the weight straight up until you are back in the starting position with control, that's one rep.

CHEST

Dumbbell Bench Press

Starting by lying on your back on a flat bench, holding a dumbbell in each hand. Bring the weight to a point just above your shoulders palms facing toward your feet and elbows out, press the weight straight up until there right over your collarbone, then slowly lower them to the starting position. Dumbbell is about control, technique and form. For beginners it will be awkward, but don't let the dumbbell sway back to-wards your head and over your face, feel the stretch in your chest muscle as you drop your elbows below the level of the bench. The reason why I choose dumbbells, is for control and technique which will also help stimulate that challenge muscle that will give you great development. Don't forget to keep your head straight and always on the bench, don't lift your butt off the bench either.

Incline Dumbbell Press

First you have to remember that incline is a little harder to do than flat bench so it's okay if you are using a smaller weight than you did for the flat bench. Sitting on an incline bench which should be in a 45 degree angle, with dumbbell in each hand place them on your thighs one at a time position them on your shoulder lean back feet flat on the ground head straight and flat on the bench, press the weight up to a point over your upper chest while you are lowering the weight down (inhale) and (exhale) bring the weight up.

Shoulders

Seated Dumbbell Press

You need to do this exercise on a shoulder bench that have back sup-port and don't lean your head back to far, look straight forward chin up, shoulders squared and stick your chest out, feet flat on the floor, dumbbell in each hand, at shoulder height, elbows out and palms facing forward press the dumbbell up and in, but do not let the weight touch above your head because that will cause stress to you joint and elbows, control the weight. Do not let it sway back and forth do not lock your arms so your arms will almost be straight when you come up, then slowly lower the dumbbell to the starting position you always want to grab a weight that you can perform good technique and form.

Bent Over Raises

By standing with your feet shoulder width apart dumbbells in each hand, bend forward your upper body should be parallel with the floor with your arms hanging straight down, palms facing each other this exercise is for your rear deltoids (delts). Do not lean over too much or bunch your back because your torso should almost be parallel with the floor, raise the dumbbell by pulling your arms apart and move your el-bows up, remember do not lift your torso when you are bringing your arms up when you get to the top with the dumbbell they should be in line with your shoulder, then slowly lower the weight back down to the starting position. Remember you should use lighter weights for good form and technique.

One Arm Dumbbell Rows

Start with your right foot flat on the floor and your left knee resting on a flat bench lean forward so you can support the weight on your upper body with your left arm on the bench, your back should be straight, head up pick the dumbbell up with your right hand concentrate on pulling your elbows as far as you can slowly lower the dumbbell back down to the starting positions. Do not hunch your back after you do the right side then do the left side with the same instructions.

Dumbbell Pullover

With a flat bench lie across with only your upper back making contact so that means that your head is slightly on the bench as well, hold the weight above your head at arm length over your face, do not raise your hips up as the dumbbell is lowed behind your head without lowering your hips, in an arch slowly inhale deep when you feel that stretch left the dumbbell back up in an arch and exhale deeply.

Arms Triceps

Dumbbell Extension (triceps)

This exercise is kind of complicates as for as grabbing the weight, early in my book I spoke about variation grip, I like to grab the dumb-bell with my right index finger and thumb then I will switch grip with my left index finger and thumb that way I can concentrate on totally on my triceps and focus of that muscle and not on trying to even my grip with the weight, holding the weight firmly and your feet are shoulder width apart, knees slightly bent to take the press off your back. Grasp one end of the dumbbell with both hands (palms up) raise the dumbbell above your head slowly lower the dumbbell behind your head, elbows close to your head focus on your triceps when pressing the weight back up you have to put a arch so you don't hit your head until your arms are slightly lock directly over your head.

Bench Dips (triceps)

Doing this exercise you have to be close to a bench because you do not want to extend to far away from the bench that will cause stress on you, do not want to lower your body to far that will cause stress also to the shoulder, position yourself on a flat bench bend your legs and place your hand on front of the bench your feet are in front of you, most of your body weight is resting on your arms, elbows always tucked against your side slowly lower your body down, your upper arms should be parallel with your shoulder while your hips are dropped straight down, then straighten your arms coming back up. Do not lean or arch your body in an angle.

Arms Biceps

Incline Dumbbell Curls (biceps)

This exercise also have to be done with a lighter weight because you do not want to put too much stress on the shoulders or rotator cuff, sit down on an incline bench with a dumbbell in each hand, back flat on the bench, head straight your shoulder squared and your chest elevated when starting, your hand should be hanging straight down, do not lean forward or swing the weights up, control with good form and technique while your back is flat against the bench and your palm are facing for-ward, curl the dumbbell and let it hang to get that full biceps stretch before you lift it back up.

Seated Dumbbell (curls)

Sitting on the edge of a flat bench arms at your side with dumbbell on each hand take a deep breath while focusing on flexing your biceps, do not lean back or forward as you lower or bring the weight up, your back supposed to be straight with your palms facing forward slowly curl both arms toward your shoulder try not to swing the weights up and try to keep your upper arms and torso still, then lower the dumbbells slowly down to the starting position feel the negative.

<u>Legs Quadriceps</u>

<u>Dumbbell Squats</u>

Holding two dumbbells that you can control with perfect form, this is an exercise you really have to be careful with, you don't want to hurt your lower back, palms facing in stand with your feet shoulder width apart while keeping your shoulder, back and head straight, bend your legs at the knee and lower your hips until your thighs are parallel to the floor lift yourself back up by pushing your heels up to the starting position keep your back as straight throughout this exercise your knees are not supposed to go pass your toes.

<u>Leg Extension (quadriceps)</u>

Sitting down on a leg extension machine and hook your ankles behind the roller pad, you should adjust the roller pad to rest on the lower part of your shin not the middle of your shin or the top of your toe and do not let your hip come up off the seat also make sure that you are lowering the weight all the way down to stretch that muscle all the way up as well it should be some handles on the machine or on the side of the seat to keep you from lifting your hips slowly lift the weight up until your leg are straightened and squeeze your quads then slowly lift the weight up until your legs are straighten and squeeze your quads then slowly lower the weight back down, remember all the way down some people go half the way which put too much stress on your knees.

Dumbbell Lunge (hamstrings)

Stand with your feet together toes pointed straight forward not pointed in or out, also get a weight that you will have control and balance, back straight, shoulders and your head is straight step forward with your foot, bend at your knees and lower your hips until your left knee is almost touching the floor push with your right leg raising yourself back up to a starting position, you can do one leg at a time then do the same amount of reps for the other leg or you can do the right leg then come up then do the left leg, whatever one you choose.

Straight Leg Deadlifts (hamstrings)

This exercise are a great exercise it will help the lower back so don't go to heavy, stand up straight with your feet shoulder width apart with dumbbells in each hand and your palm are facing toward your legs, bend forward at the hip and slowly lower the dumbbell in front of you until the weight almost touch the floor, your back supposed to be straight throughout the exercise, while concentrating on the muscles in the back of your legs (hamstrings) raise your upper body and the weight to the starting position, do not hunch over keep your back straight.

Standing Calf Raises (calves)

Use a calf raise machine position yourself that the ball of your feet are on the platform and the pad with the weight is on your shoulder, do not put so much weight on the machine that you are hunching your back, when doing this exercise do not bend at your hips or knees, keep your back straight shoulder squared and your face forward, slowly lower the weight down, feel the stretch then lift the weight up as high as you can hold the contraction for 1 or 2 seconds.

Seated Calf Raises (calves)

They also have a calf raise machine, if not you can use 2 dumbbells in each hand, your feet should be shoulder width apart and raise as high as you can and hold for 1 to 2 seconds, but let's talk about the calf raise machine, with the ball of your feet on the platform and the knee pad is on the lower part of your knees, slowly lower your heels and let your calf muscle stretch as far down as you can, bring the weight up as high as you can and squeeze at the top then lower the weight back down.

Anaerobic Exercises are done on:
Monday, Wednesday, and Friday

Aerobic Exercises are done on:
Tuesday, Thursday, and Saturday

MONDAY:	SETS	REPS
Dumbbell Bench Press (chest)	3	10.10.10
Incline Dumbbell Press (chest)	3	10.10.10
One Arm Dumbbell Row (back)	3	10.10.10
Dumbbell Pullover (back)	3	12.10.8
Seated Dumbbell Press (shoulders)	3	10.10.10
Bend Over Raises (shoulders)	3	10.8.8

TUESDAY:

(Jogging outdoor, or on a treadmill for 20 to 30 mins, then do your Ad workout)

	SETS	REPS
Hanging Leg Raise	3	10.10.10
Hanging Oblique Crunch	3	10 per side
Rope Crunch	3	15.15.15
Knee In	3	15.15.15
Exercise Ball Crunch	3	15.15.15

WEDNESDAY:	SETS	REPS
Incline Dumbbell Curl (biceps)	4	10.10.10
Seated Dumbbell Curl (biceps)	4	10.10.10
Dumbbell Extensions (triceps)	4	10.10.10
Bench Dips (triceps)	4	10.10.10

THURSDAY:

(Jogging outdoor, or on a treadmill for 20 to 30 mins, then do your Ad workout)

Hanging Leg Raise	3	10.10.10
Hanging Oblique Crunch	3	10 per side
Rope Crunch	3	15.15.15
Knee In	3	15.15.15
Exercise Ball Crunch	3	15.15.15

FRIDAY:

Dumbbell Squat (legs)	3	10.10.10
Leg Extensions	3	12.10.10
Leg Press	3	12.10.10
Dumbbell Lunge (legs)	3	10.10.10
Straight Legs Deadlifts (hamstrings)	3	10.10.10
Standing Calf Raise (calves)	3	15.12.10
Seated Calf Raises (calves)	3	15.12.10

SATURDAY:

(Jogging outdoor, or on a treadmill for 20 to 30 mins, then do your Ab workout)

Hanging Leg Raise	3	10.10.10
Hanging Oblique Crunch	3	10 per side
Rope Crunch	3	15.15.15
Knee In	3	15.15.15
Exercise Ball Crunch	3	15.15.15

SUNDAY IS REST DAY

Tips for ABS

To get the best results for training your abdominals, or walking, swimming, running, these exercises should be done early in the morning be-fore you eat. Schedule 20 or 35 minutes for abdominal exercise, rather than throwing it in at the end of your weight training. This way you can get the best results.

Do not twist too much at the waist; it may cause spinal disc injury. Further, doing too much bending and twisting can make your waist wider, not thinner, by making those muscles bigger. When doing abs exercise do them in a slow controlled motion so you can get at the deep fibers of your stomach.

For Women:

Lower abdominal crunches	10 to 15 Reps
Side Crunches	10 to 15 Reps
Lying Crunches	10 to 15 Reps
Rope Lying Crunches	10 to 15 Reps

Chapter 8

Workout with The Bar

The bar workout can play an important part in shaping your physique with variation grip it will complement the shoulder (anterior, medial, and posterior) Back (upper and mid back muscles and latissimus dorsi) that will create a powerful V-shaped torso, also making your waist look smaller plus helps your biceps. I have to admit that technology and the way we workout today have changed since the 50's and 60's.

Doing the bar behind the neck or doing shoulder press behind the neck that training principles are debatable even though it will help the upper and other regions of the lats, you will risk hurting your rotator cuffs, but it is other choices of variation grip that can help stimulated certain muscle by doing the bar. Take hold of the chinning bar, then pull yourself up try to touch the top of your chest to the bar, if not try to bring your chin above the bar hold for a brief moment, then lower yourself back to the starting position now don't lock at your arms because that can cause undue stress to your elbow joints, but you can ex-tend them before you go back up. These are the variation grip I have learned in my own experience of working out, but remember you want to use great technique and form in doing the bar.

Overhand Grip

Shoulder Width:

Helps your upper back also develops shoulder girdle and lats.

Close-In:

With hands 6ins apart help forearm, posterior (rear deltoids) mid back

Close-In:

With triangle device or you can put your right hand in front of the other but then you should put your left hand grip on the next set, but this helps develops those little fingers that lies under the outside of the pec, (serratus anterior).

Underhand Grip or Reverse Grip

Shoulder Width:

Develop the upper lats and back

Close-In:

With your hands 6ins apart to develop the serratior anterior in the lower lats.

Mix Grip:

Develop a powerful V-Shape torso also help the biceps. Doing mix grip on the bar: Put your right hand in the front, first set then you would put your left hand first on the second sets.

<u>Remember</u>

Doing the triangle device or placing on hand in front of the other, as you pull yourself up slightly lean your head back so that your chest would touch your hand or almost touch your hand. If you are using the bar without the triangle device you have to do an even number of sets because you have to switch right hand to left the left hand to right hand.

With the mix grip you have to do is switch overhand with an even number of sets so if you do the right hand overhand you would do the left hand underhand then you would change to your right hand under-hand and your left overhand. You can intensify your bar workout by adds some weight to your exercise but I recommend that when you have advance in the bar workout.

<u>The Bar, Dips, and Push-Up Exercise</u>

This workout is going to be intense because your body has to adapt to this circuit training exercise or you can say triple set workout. It consists of several exercises back to back, with no rest in between. 10 reps of the bar, 10 reps of dips and 10 reps of push-ups then rest for 60 seconds, that's one set. When you get advanced in this workout you intensify this exercise with weight on the bar and dips, switch your pushup (without weights) Incline, decline and diamond like push-ups. This is how you do diamond push-ups, you would get in a regular push -up position, shape your trigger fingers and thumbs like a diamond but you should bring them as close as you possibly can. With each variation grip of the bar you are doing sets with dips and push-ups that will come to a total of 12 sets of bar 12 sets of dips and 12 sets of push-ups.

> 2 Sets Overhand Grip (shoulder width)
>
> 2 Sets Close-in Overhand Grip (6ins apart)
>
> 2 Sets With the triangle device or one hand in front of the other
>
> 2 Sets Under hand or Reverse Grip (shoulder width)
>
> 2 Sets Close-in under hand or Reverse Grip (6ins apart)
>
> 2 Sets Mix Grips

Chapter 9

30 Days to a Killer Core

<u>Double Your Strength</u>

1. To do squats, keep your back straight, knees bent, toes straight ahead, and feet hip width apart. Lift the bar off the rack. When your quads are parallel to the floor, explode up using your quads, hamstrings, glutes, and keep your back straight and head up. Find a weight that you can do 5 sets of 6 reps.

2. Get into a squatting position with the bar centered over the balls of your feet. Grip the bar with an overhanded-underhanded grip. Pull the bar straight up with your legs and back, keeping it close to your body. As it passes your knees, arch backwards, carefully lowering the weight keeping your eyes forward so you won't hunch over. Find a weight that you can do 4 set of 5 reps.

3. Get two flat benches, one that you can put your hand on, and ex-tend your legs onto the other one, suspending yourself by your heels. Put a weight on your lap, lower your upper body until your elbows are at a 90 degree angle. Make sure that the weight doesn't slide off. Keep your elbows close to your body and raise your upper body back up into the starting position. Find a weight that you can do 3 sets of 10 reps.

Simple Exercise Routine:

Exercise:	Set	Reps
Squats (legs)	1	10 to 15
Bent- Over row (back)	1	10 to 15
Bench Press (chest0	1	10 to 15
Barbell Curls (arms)	1	10 to 15
Crunches (abs)	1	10 to 15
Dumbbell Presser (delts)	1	10 to 15

Do 10 reps of wide grip push-ups, followed immediately by 10 with a narrow grip with your thumbs and forefingers touching in a diamond. Doing this works the shoulders, chest and triceps- The Three Major Muscles Groups.

Recuperation

You train because you want to get big, and essentially the muscle building process occurs in the following three stages: Stimulation, Recovery, and Growth.

The stimulation stage is accomplished by putting training stress on the body, then begins the recovery phase. Once the recovery phase is complete, muscle growth occurs. Only after muscle growth has taken place then it's time to train those particular muscles again.

Over training (Symptoms & Cures)

Generally feeling tired
Irritable
Trouble sleeping
Loss of appetite
Joint aches
Light headed and nausea
Not being in a positive frame of mind

I realized that improvement is enhanced not by training harder and longer, but by training smarter. Think smart and recuperate to accumulate.

Eating whole foods rich in protein and essential fats, as well as cards like sweet potatoes, brown rice, and whole grain breads whenever possible.

Shrug Behind the Back

With feet shoulder width apart, knees slightly bent, extend your arms fully and press your shoulders as high as possible. Squeeze your tri- ceps for a count or two, then return to the start position.

Reverse EZ Bar Curl

Calves, traps and forearm all respond well to high rep training, so lighten the weight. Try to do 2 set 30 reps.

Leg Workout: (reverse the routine)

	Sets	Reps
Squats	3	15 to 20
Leg Press	3	15 to 20
Leg Extension	3	15 to 20
Lying Leg Curls	3	15 to 20
Standing Calf Raises	3	20
Seated Calf Raises	3	20

Chest Workout: Sets Reps

	Sets	Reps
1. Incline Barbell Press	3	12 to 15
Dumbbell Bench Press	3	12 to 15
Incline Dumbbell Fly	3	15
2. Incline Dumbbell Fly	3	15
Barbell bench Press	3	12 to 15
Incline Barbell Press	3	12 to 15

After a 4 minute warm-up jog around the track, take off for a 20 second sprint, and then a 10 second rest, and so on until those unpleasant 4 minute are up. Then close it out with another 4 minute jog around the track to cool down.

The 4 D's

DESIRE: YOU MUST WANT IT

DETERMINATION: TO DEVELOP A GOAL WITH ACCOMPLISHMENT

DISCIPLINE: YOUR MIND MUST BE INTO SCULPTING A PERFECT PHYSIQUE

DEDICATION: WHEN YOU WANT IT BADLY ENOUGH

Taking caffeine about 30 to 45 minutes before cardio-workout can increase the fat- burning process.

First warm-up, then do 1 or 2 sets, then go to your max and decrease the weight

Flat Bench Dumbbell Press 3 sets of 15, 20, 10

Incline Dumbbell Press 3 sets of 15, 12, 10

Training Split

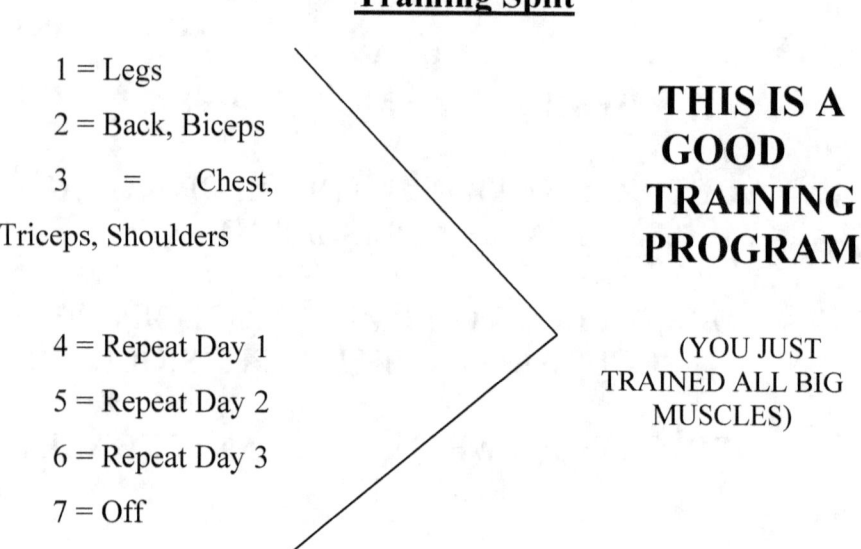

1 = Legs

2 = Back, Biceps

3 = Chest, Triceps, Shoulders

4 = Repeat Day 1

5 = Repeat Day 2

6 = Repeat Day 3

7 = Off

THIS IS A GOOD TRAINING PROGRAM

(YOU JUST TRAINED ALL BIG MUSCLES)

Straight Leg Crunch = Perform crunches with your knees straight and your feet pointed towards the ceiling.

Front Barbell Raise

Back Exercises

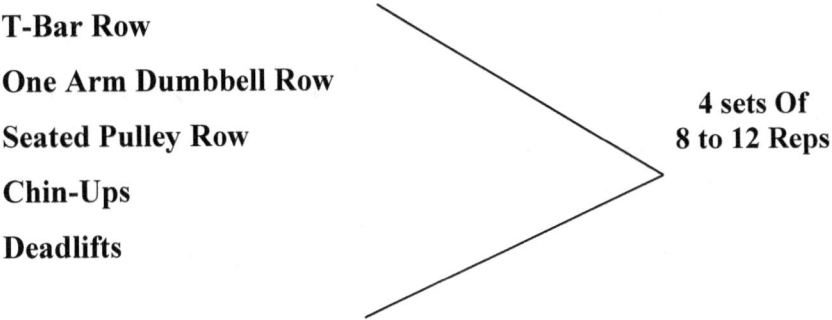

T-Bar Row

One Arm Dumbbell Row

Seated Pulley Row

Chin-Ups

Deadlifts

**4 sets Of
8 to 12 Reps**

Share your passion and try to instill in others the habits of going to the gym on a regular basis!

Exercise:

CURL WORKOUT	SETS	REPS
Standing Barbell Curl	4	15 ,12, 10, 10
Standing EZ Bar Spider Curl (Hanging your arms straight down from your shoulders)	4	15, 12, 10, 6-8
Alternating Dumbbell Hammer Curl	4	10,12
Seated Alternating Dumbbell Curl	4	10, 8, 8, 6-8

LEG WORKOUT	SETS	REPS
Leg Extensions	2	25
Barbell Squats	4	8, 10
Romanian Deadlift	4	8, 10
Leg Press	4	50
Hack Squat	4	50

STRENGTH GAINS

Perform a set of deadlifts for 6 to 8 reps, rest 2 minutes then perform a set of dumbbell bench press for another 6 to 8 reps, then rest again. Then repeat both exercised twice more for a total of 3 supersets. The heavy weight will promote strength gains, while the switching be-tween lower and upper body work will create a state of "turbulence" in the body, confusing your metabolism so it won't be likely to store bulk on your frame.

THE LUNGE MATRIX

With your right leg, perform a lunge to the front, then to the side, and then on a 45 angle behind you, and to the left. That's on rep, perform 3 sets of 4 reps in each direction for both legs, resting 30 – 45 seconds between sets.

THE CROSSOVER LUNGE

From the starting position, cross your left leg over your right, and lunge as far as you can to your right side, landing on your heel. To ease the pressure on your front knee, land with your foot at a 45 angle. Perform 3 sets of 12 reps on each side, resting 90 seconds be-tween sets. Do this exercise at the start of your leg workout.

"The Pain is Temporary, The Pride is Forever"

Lift for Failure

Complete failure is more than just stopping when the weight feels too heavy. Complete failure comes only when you have tapped into your hidden reserve of will and strength - and it may come a rep or two after your muscles tell you it's time to pack up and go home. A strong mind will always beat the body, no matter how strong the body is. Going to total failure is a great way to stimulate muscle growth.

How much progress you make in this program involves a lot of things you can't control, like muscle length, number of fast twitch fi-ber (not slow-twitch fiber). Neural efficiency and the things that fall under the category of genetics. However, there are a lot of things you can control. As I pointed out, muscle cells don't live in a vacuum-they're a part of you and share whatever mistreatment you subject yourself to. Consistency is also vital.

Take Aspirin

Studies show that taking regular doses of aspirin, especially if you have a history of heart or circulation problems, offers significant protection from strokes. Aspirin helps keep arteries from clogging up and blocking blood flow to the brain or heart. It takes only small doses of aspirin to obtain these benefits. We're talking 30 to 81 milligrams, or breaking a standard 325 milligram pill into quarters will give you four correct doses. (Check with your doctor before starting an aspirin regimen), but if he agrees, then an 81 milligram does every day or every other day is beneficial.

30 MINUTE WORKOUT
(Upper Body Circuit)

Do one set of an exercise, then immediately move to the next; upper body blast in a minimal amount of time. Also when you want to add a cardiovascular element to your lifting as you take almost no rest be-tween sets. Each muscle groups rests while the others are trained.

MUSCLE GROUP	EXERCISE	SETS	REPS
Chest	Incline Barbell Press	1	8
Back	Bent Over Barbell Row	1	8
Shoulders	Arnold Press (Dumbbell)	1	8
Biceps	Incline Dumbbell	1	8
Triceps	Overhead Dumbbell Extension	1	8
Chest	Smith- Machine Press	1	10
Back (traps)	Barbell Shrug	1	10
Shoulders	Cable Front Raise	1	10
Biceps	Barbell Curl	1	10
Triceps	Dip	1	10
Back	Straight Arm Pull down	1	15
Chest	Cable Crossover	1	15
Shoulders	Bent Over Lateral Raise	1	15
Biceps	EZ Bar Preacher	1	15
Triceps	Two Arm Dumbbell Kickback	1	15

30 Minute Workout

(Whole Body Timed)

You'll simply do as many reps as you can in five minutes, resting when you need to. You will probably get fatigue quickly, and will be working off the rest. For each exercise select a weight that will cause you to fail at 10 reps. Do 10 reps right off the bat, then rest until you feel ready to go again. Do as many reps as you can, then rest again. Do this for five minutes, which means you'll have to keep a close eye on the clock or your watch. If you end up going too light or too heavy, don't bother repeating a set, which could extend your gym time. Just make a note for your next go around. Another good rule of thumb is to perform 1 – 2 warm up sets on each body part.

MUSCLE GROUP	EXERCISE	TIME
Chest	Chest Press Machine	5 mins
Legs	Leg Press	5 mins
Shoulders	Lateral Raise Machine	5 mins
Back	Lat Pulldown or Seated Row	5 mins
Triceps	Cable Pressdown	5 mins
Biceps	Machine Preacher Curl	5 mins

30 Minute Workout

(Upper Body Pre-Exhaust)

An upper body only routine that incorporates a bit of the pre-exhaust principle into back, chest, and shoulders, and one set of 100 reps each for triceps and biceps. The target muscle group will give out first since its pre-exhaust, and the 100 rep set will shock your bi's and tri's in a hurry. Make sure you do the chest, shoulder, and back exercise in order – the single joint moves before the multi-joint ones. You can swap the order of bi's and tri's, and abs.

MUSCLE GROUP	EXERCISE	SETS	REPS
Chest	Cable Crossover	2	15, 20
	Flat Bench Dumbbell Press	3	6, 8, 12
Shoulders	Dumbbell Lateral Raise	2	15,20
	Seated Overhead Dumbbell Press	3	6, 8, 12
Back	Straight Arm Pull-down	2	15, 20
	Bent Over Barbell Row	3	6, 8, 12
Triceps	Cable Pull-down	1	100
Biceps	Barbell Curl	1	100
Abs	Hanging Knee Raise	1	20

30 Minutes Workout

(At home legs + Chest + Abs)

A routine for the quads, glutes, hams, pecs, calves, and abs that you can do at home with no equipment except an exercise ball. Rest 30 seconds between sets, except when going from hamstrings to calves, calves to chest, and chest to abs, where no rest in necessary.

MUSCLE GROUP	EXERCISE	SETS	REPS/TIME
Quads	Wall Squats	2	45-60 secs
	Sissy Squats	2	10
Hamstrings	Exercise Ball	2	10
	Leg Curls	2	10
Calves	Standing Calf Raise	3	20
Chest	Decline Push Ups	2	12
	Standing Push Ups	2	10
Abs	Crunch	1	20
	Reverse Crunch	1	20
	Double Crunch	1	20

Dealing
With
Chronic Diseases

Chapter 10

Dealing with Chronic Diseases

Before considering training a person with a chronic disorder, the first and most important thing is that you are qualified to help the client in his or her current condition. You need to discuss with your physician information including medical history, all medications the client ingest and their impact of the training process.

Arthritis

Osteoarthritis:

Is a progressive form of arthritis, the damage to the joint surface is progressive and irreversible, OA sufferers also experience constant pain.

Rheumatoid (RA):

Is seen in the distal joints, such as fingers, and knees. Both can interfere with the normal range of motion.

Obesity

Most obese people become obese from trying to lose weight the wrong way, typically by "Yo-Yo dieting", over 40% of the U.S population is obese. Obesity is determined by the percentage of body fat. For women, obesity begins at 32% body fat. For men Obesity begins at 25% body fat.

Diabetes

There are 2 forms of diabetes

Type 1- Insulin dependent, and is commonly referred to as juvenile onset diabetes. The client is forced to take insulin injections on a regular basis.

Type 2- Referred to as non-insulin dependent or maturity onset diabetes. This form is commonly a result of obesity and may be treated successfully with diet modifications and exercise. As they lose weight, Type 2 diabetics may experience some lower level of symptoms.

With either type of diabetes, it is a good idea to check your insulin levels before and after exercise to avoid severe swings in blood glucose levels. These changes can appear for up to 4 to 6 hours an exercise session. To compensate for this training effect, it may be necessary for the diabetic to take smaller dosage of insulin or to increase carbohydrate intake before the onset of exercise. For persons with either form of arthritis, weight bearing exercise may not be the best choice for exercise. Instead, water exercise or stationary bicycling may provide them with the greatest relief.

Additional Resources

Drop Pounds, Not Calories

We all want to cut a trim profile around the middle. A lean physique looks better, and more youthful, than a pear shaped one. To stay slim, however, men mistakenly tend to cut back on calories when the real villain is lack of exercise, and to much fat. In fact, trying to keep weight off simple by cutting calories may not be a smart idea. By eating less you risk cheating your body of important nutrients, for healthy weight loss is to exercise more. (As you reach middle age you need to eat more calories as well. Just be sure they're low fat calories. As a rule of thumb, 60 to 70 percent of your diet should consist of foods high in complex carbohydrates, such as breads, pasta, and beans.)

Muscle Fiber Twitches

Your body has approximately a quarter billion skeletal muscle fibers. All of which can be categorized as three skeletal muscle tissue fibers which have different support systems in capillaries the white fast twitch muscle fibers have few capillaries and is very strong but cannot function very long. The red fast twitch muscle fibers have more capillaries than the white but, not as strong as the white. Lastly the red slow twitch fibers have a tremendous number of capillaries allowing for long term sustained activity, with very little strength.

Breathe

The correct way to breathe while performing an exercise is to exhale while you are forcing the weight up (concentric muscle contractions) and to inhale while you are lowering the weight (eccentric the negative). If you are bench pressing you exhale while you are pushing the weight up and inhale when you are lowering the weight down to your chest.

Stretching

Stretch and warm up before training also after training here are some stretching exercises you can do for your muscles. You need to hold all stretching positions for at least 5 seconds.

Chest Stretching:

By grabbing a pole with one arm at a time, slowly turn away from the pole and allow your arms to be as far behind the body as possible, do not overextend your chest.

Back Stretching:

By grabbing a pole with both arms bending your knees and sitting back in order to fully extend your arms which you would feel this stretch in your lats and lower back.

Shoulder Stretching:

By grabbing one of your triceps with the opposite hand without moving your torso, pull your arms as far as possible then repeat with the other arm.

Thigh Stretching:

By grabbing a pole with one arm and bending the opposite leg bring your foot towards your butt, with your free hand holding your ankle, slowly lift your foot as comfortable as possible, then repeat with the other leg.

Hamstring Stretching:

By stepping forward with your left heel while bending your right knee, keep your left leg straight and toes pointed up. By placing your hand on your left thigh, bend forward at the waist and feel the stretch in your hamstrings.

Calves Stretching:

By grabbing a pole with both arms stand on a raised surface and placing one foot on the edge of the surface in order to allow your heels to go down as far as comfortable, and then do the other leg.

I recommend that you do the stretching exercise before and after you work that muscle.

Training
Diary

Day 1:

Warm-Up:

Body Part (Exercise)	Set	Rep	Weight

Cardio

Nutrition:
Breakfast

Snack

Lunch

Snack

Dinner

Water Intake:

Day 2:

Warm-Up:

Body Part (Exercise)	Set	Rep	Weight

Cardio

Nutrition:
Breakfast

Snack

Lunch

Snack

Dinner

Water Intake:

Day 3:

Warm-Up:

Body Part (Exercise)	Set	Rep	Weight

Cardio

Nutrition:
Breakfast

Snack

Lunch

Snack

Dinner

Water Intake:

Day 4:

Warm-Up:

Body Part (Exercise)	Set	Rep	Weight

Cardio

Nutrition:
Breakfast

Snack

Lunch

Snack

Dinner

Water Intake:

Day 5:

Warm-Up:

Body Part (Exercise)	Set	Rep	Weight

Cardio

Nutrition:
Breakfast

Snack

Lunch

Snack

Dinner

Water Intake:

Day 6:

Warm-Up:

Body Part (Exercise)	Set	Rep	Weight

Cardio

Nutrition:
Breakfast

Snack

Lunch

Snack

Dinner

Water Intake:

Day 7:

Warm-Up:

Body Part (Exercise)	Set	Rep	Weight

Cardio

Nutrition:
Breakfast

Snack

Lunch

Snack

Dinner

Water Intake:

Day 8:

Warm-Up:

Body Part (Exercise)	Set	Rep	Weight

Cardio

Nutrition:
Breakfast

Snack

Lunch

Snack

Dinner

Water Intake:

Day 9:

Warm-Up:

Body Part (Exercise)	Set	Rep	Weight

Cardio

Nutrition:
Breakfast

Snack

Lunch

Snack

Dinner

Water Intake:

Day 10:

Warm-Up:

Body Part (Exercise)	Set	Rep	Weight

Cardio

Nutrition:
Breakfast

Snack

Lunch

Snack

Dinner

Water Intake:

Glossary

Aerobic: (Requiring Oxygen) metabolism occurs during low intensity, long duration exercise, like walking, running and bike riding

Anaerobic: (Without Oxygen) metabolism in muscle tissue occurs during intense physical activities like weight training The glossary terms are often set off in some way, using a bold or italic font. It is also common to set off the entries with a hanging indent and/or extra space between the terms.

Atrophy: A decrease in size of muscle tissue from lack of use

Body Composition: The percentage of your body weight composed of fat compared to fat free mass

Carbohydrates: Organic compounds containing carbon, hydrogen, and oxygen. Very effective fuel source for the body

Calories: The unit for measuring the energy value of food

Cholesterol: Known as a bad fat, there are different types of cholesterol, DHL and LDL, (HDL being the "GOOD" for and LDL being the "BAD" form

Concentric: The lifting phase of an exercise
Density: Helps maintain and keeps the bone stronger when you get up in age

Diet: Food and drink regularly consumed by a person

Deficiency: A suboptimal level of one or more nutrients that are essential for good health

Eccentric: The lower phase of an exercise

Fat: Calories of all the macronutrient, there are two types of fat: saturated fats "bad" and unsaturated fats "good"

Glycogen: Stored form of carbohydrates energy that is reserved in muscle

Lactic Acid: By product created by a lack of oxygen flow to the working muscle. Lactic acid is created by anaerobic activities such as weight training exercise. It is believed that its presence cause a surge in growth hormone levels

Testosterone: Hormone responsible for increasing muscle size. Even though this hormone is predominantly present in males, it is also present in women to a lesser degree. It is believed that this hormone also aids in fat loss to a lesser degree

Metabolism: The rate at which the body utilized calories and nutrients in order to sustain its daily activities

Protein: Are the building block of muscles, enzymes, and some hormones

Saturated Fats: "Bad Fats" contain no open spots on their carbon skeleton

Supplements: Are used to help you achieve optimal nutrient intake

Unsaturated Fats: "Good Fats" The main source of these fats are from plant food, sunflower, and flaxseed oils

Vitamins: Organic compounds that are vital to life